OPTIMIZE LIFE FOR YOUR AGING PARENTS AND YOU

PAULA EDWARDS BERRYANN

outskirtspress

DENVER, COLORADO

Outskirts Press, Inc.
http://www.outskirtspress.com

ISBN: 978-1-4327-9738-6

Outskirts Press and the "OP" logo are trademarks belonging to Outskirts Press, Inc.

PRINTED IN THE UNITED STATES OF AMERICA

Dedicated to my loving and special parents,
Paul Lemmon and Catherine Erline (Orr) Edwards

Ephesians 6:2-3 *"Honor your father and mother"* **(this is the first commandment with a promise)**, *"that it may be well with you and that you may live long on earth."*

Deuteronomy 5:16 *"Honor your father and your mother, as the Lord your God commanded you; that your days may be prolonged, and that it may go well with you, in the land which the Lord your God gives you."*

Exodus 20:12 *"Honor your father and your mother, that your days may be long in the land which the Lord your God gives you."*

The Bible tells us the important things more than once!

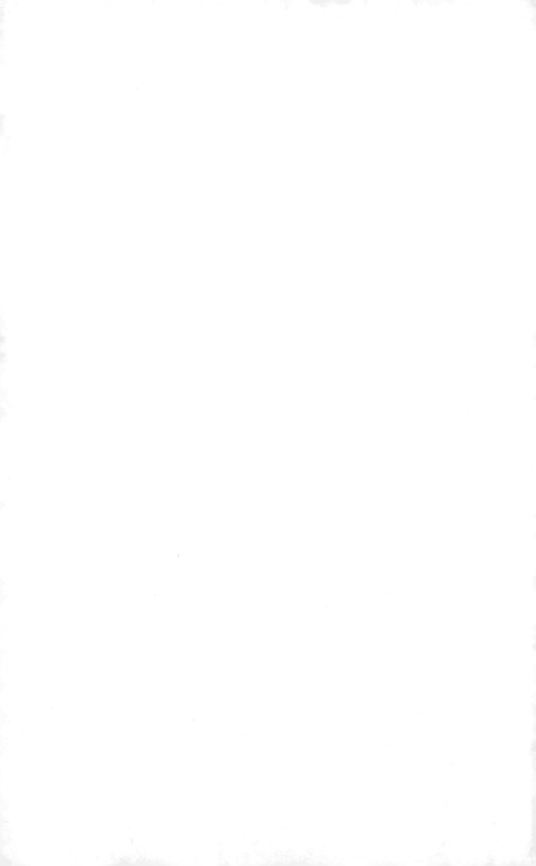

Table of Contents

Introduction

This book is intended as a "to do" checklist to help you and your parents.

Having aging parents is difficult, new territory for us Baby Boomers.

Do not let your parents ruin your health, your marriage, or your life.

You have to take care of yourself in order to take care of others.

The goal is for you to outlive your parents. Do not let your parents' aging age you!

Change happens. People fear change because the result is unknown, and life might get worse. The **goal** is to make change be as positive as possible.

Aging is a transition through the phases of life: childhood, adolescence, emerging adulthood, adulthood, active retirement, and old age. Death is certain.

This book is intended to give you things to consider in dealing with aging parents and optimizing the quality of life for your parents and you. Only you know the correct choices for your parents, you, your spouse, and your siblings. Those choices can change as the circumstances change.

If you are married, there could be four parents who become your responsibility. If your parents or in-laws divorced and remarried, there could be more adults who need you to be their caregivers. You might need to assist your parents' siblings or your siblings through their senior years.

I am an individual dealing with aging parents and have observed other friends and relatives helping their parents. I have not done everything right, but I hope you can learn from reviewing my choices. My **goal** is that my experience and insight in this book will save you at least one headache and one heart ache! I want to help others as they provide care for their parents and relatives. My aim is that you know about your parents' assets to make their golden years as happy as possible.

A later section of this book, **Lessons to Learn**, includes items to consider in your personal dealing with aging. Hopefully these can make it easier on you, your children, and caregivers.

This book is not intended to provide medical or legal advice. You will need to consult doctors, counselors, lawyers, and accountants for their professional advice. I am not a professionally trained internist, psychologist, estate lawyer, or CPA.

People are living longer. We do not know how long our parents will live. Mom is 91 and could live one week or ten years. Actress Betty White is still active and vibrant at 90.

Do not assume you personally can care for your parents their entire lives.

In the business world we are accustomed to investigating problems, making decisions, taking actions, getting closure, and moving on to the next project. At work you are usually in control of your choices. But relationships and dealing with aging parents are not like straightforward projects at work. This responsibility does not end until both of your parents die, their estates are settled, and their house is sold. With people living longer that could mean you take care of them longer than they took care of you! When dealing with aging parents you are not in charge, your good ideas of needed change are not readily accepted, and your parents want to keep the status quo. As their health and faculties decline, changes are inevitable. The information I present is to give you things to consider, so you can review choices and have plans ready when needed. You want the changes to occur in a positive direction without panic or crisis.

Parents have been responsible, independent adults. Losing control of their lives is a difficult process. Many will fight you about any changes. They do not like the deterioration of their minds and bodies. Depending on your relationship with your parents and their amount of flexibility, this period of time can be extremely difficult for you and them or can hopefully improve your relationship. Their reactions, choices, and attitudes, however, might make your job harder.

Some parents are sensitive to the amount of work required by their children for their care and do what makes things easier for the children. Some, like Mom, never did think about that perspective or viewpoint and, without realizing it, did not make things easy for me.

This could be a ride on an emotional roller coaster. My intent in writing this book is to:

- Minimize your mental and physical pain by thinking before action is required.
- Know when it is time for you to become the parent and take control.
- Help you do the right things for your parents.
- Minimize financial impacts on your parents and you.
- Hopefully improve your relationship with your parents.

It is a hard decision to move your parents out of their home. They can never go back. It is the start of a declining, difficult path to the end.

The goal of several girlfriends in dealing with their mothers was to "finish well." I am using the same goal in dealing with my aging mother.

Finish well. That is my hope for you in writing this book.

Note: For ease of discussion I will use the plural "parents" and "they."

1

Respect

Always honor your parents and be respectful of them. Their love created you, and they raised you by providing food, clothing, support, and love to get you where you are today. I love and respect Mom and my deceased father, who did an excellent job of raising me through childhood and young adulthood.

To honor my parents, their sacrifices for freedom, and lifelong accomplishments, I compiled Daddy's almost 700 letters to his wife (my mother) into a book. The smile on Mom's face at the book signing in her hometown was priceless when she celebrated her shining moment of fame as the inspiration for those letters.

Two dear family friends thought so much of my mother that they named their daughters Catherine, in honor of her. One dear friend named her son Paul, after my father.

Never forget their sacrifices for you. Many times our parents did without, so we would have opportunities, such as dentist visits, a special prom dress, college, etc. Always keep this in mind.

Remember, our parents were raised during the Depression, so many were needy growing up. In Mom's case she clings to her possessions for her identity. This generation is frugal with their money; that is why many of them are financially sound. Be sensitive to their views on money and life.

They still need a sense of accomplishment and self-worth. One friend's 95-year-old mother-in-law needs to wash the breakfast dishes daily to give her a sense of self-worth. At 88 Mom was so upset when I started paying her bills; it took away her meaning and purpose. Allow them to keep doing something, if possible, so they feel worthwhile. It also fills their time which passes so slowly.

When you help other people, it helps you more. Mom's unofficial job in her fifties and sixties was to help family and friends through their senior years. She took her mother almost daily for three years to feed her dad his supper at the nursing home. Her mother never drove and never moved to a nursing home but needed other help. Mom paid her bills, took her to doctors' appointments, ran errands, and took her shopping many times per month for over 20 years. Mom's younger brother bought Grandma's groceries weekly, provided cooked meals, and assisted in other ways, too.

When their family friend who was a childless widow needed help, Mom assisted her. When Grandpa's bachelor cousin, a World War I decorated hero, grew feeble, Mom ran his errands. When Mom's uncle had to move to a nursing home, Mom took care of his business and his needs for many years. He died at 92. These people either never drove or no longer could. She paid their bills, ran their errands, bought them groceries, filled out their forms for medical expenses and insurance, and took them to doctors' appointments.

When Mom's older brother, who never drove, needed assistance, Mom paid his bills and ran errands for him. Mom's younger brother bought his groceries and provided cooked meals while Tom lived at their family home for almost 20 years. My cousin was also very helpful to her uncle. Tom lived in a skilled care facility for about four years and died two years ago at 92.

An elderly neighbor had lost her two children in their youth. Her son played football with Daddy in high school, so she adopted our family, or we adopted her. We knew when she raised her curtain each morning that she was okay. She was very independent, but my parents helped her with anything she needed and treated her special by giving her flowers on Mother's Day and having an annual neighborhood bridge party in honor of her birthday.

Mom's faithful efforts for many years in serving and helping others along with her husband through their senior years rewarded her with a very blessed life.

Mom did for others, and now it is my turn to do for her.

2

Parents' Finances

Parents' minds can go at any time; you need to know their available resources.

Goal: Providing care for your parents and eventually having their funerals are expensive, so you need to understand what assets they own.

It might seem greedy or crass to put this topic second, but you never know when your parents' memory will be impacted, or they might have a stroke, so **immediately** collect the information listed farther down in this section. You will need to know and have access to their assets to properly care for your parents, but they will only provide this information if they trust you.

You need to know their finances to plan their future. They will fight you about this — it is their personal information; they are in charge. They will accuse you of wanting to steal their money, but it is critical and imperative you know this information! Prescriptions, doctors' bills, health insurance, physical therapy, assisted living, skilled care facilities, and funerals are very expensive.

You need to understand their financial status before selecting their next living quarters and planning for their future care.

Mom never did summarize her assets, but fortunately all the

necessary documents were in her safety deposit box or lockbox.

Her older brother did not summarize his assets; I had to go through every scrap of paper in two closets literally piled to the ceiling and his bedroom to identify anything important. I did find stubs from several life insurance policies, several thousand dollars in cash in envelopes and shoe boxes, and coins in small bottles! He had several mini-safes I had to force open to find money. That was money needed for his skilled care facility, doctors' bills, prescriptions, personal items, and eventually his funeral. I did not directly benefit from these findings, but at least the assets were kept in the family.

Grandma kept her treasures and important documents in the cedar chest and the secretary. The older generation even kept money in coffee cans in the basement, so I recommend you check every item in a house before selling it. In her uncle's house Mom found diamond earrings wrapped in paper in a guest room trash can and money behind pictures. Check the pockets of every item of clothing before donating or discarding. I've even heard of someone sewing money into the lining of a purse or coat.

Remember, you need to take care of their money, so it will last to take care of their needs. In the best case scenario, you will not have to use your money for their care. There might even be some left as a reward for the care you provided them through their senior years.

Costs of Assisted Living/Skilled Care Facility

It is imperative that you understand your parents' finances before decisions are made about their living facilities.

Mom's macular degeneration, diabetes, and dementia resulted in her moving into assisted living at 86, where she lived for four and a half years. She has been in a skilled care facility for almost two years. With longevity in her family she could live one month or ten years.

It is easy to spend $60,000 per year on one parent in a skilled care facility. Mom's assisted living in a small, Midwest town cost over

$22,000 per year. Her skilled care facility in that same town costs over $57,000 per year. It consists of a flat fee which includes everything except cable, so there are no surprises. This is the nicest facility in her hometown, but facilities in cities can be significantly higher. One skilled care facility in St. Louis costs $77,000 per year. Several years ago one person paid almost $80,000 per year to have 24 hour in-home care for her parents. Then you add the cost of their many medicines. Because Mom still owns her house, it costs several thousand dollars per year. One friend had both of her parents in a facility in my town; it was costing over $100,000 per year. It might not double the rate if your parents can live together in the same room, but it will cost more for food and services. Sometimes each parent requires a different level of care; for instance, one needs a memory care unit, and the other only needs independent care or assisted living.

Mom's prescriptions are over $2,000 per year beyond what the insurance covers.

Her Medicare supplemental insurance just increased $53 per month to $311.

Check potential facilities and costs where you live and where your parents live now.

Daddy had great foresight and worked an additional 5 years in an Executive role to get Mom a second retirement income. Fortunately for Mom and me, she has good pensions and savings. It is such a comfort to know she will not outlive her money.

I hope your parents are financially sound to pay the cost of their care. The enormous cost of skilled care facilities and prescriptions can drain the family nest egg and the assets from their home sale quickly. Several people in Mom's church and her facility have lived to over 100!

Locate and Organize Important Documents

Are your parents Veterans? If so, look for their discharge papers and dog tags to get their service number. Check with the Veterans

Administration to verify if they are entitled to assistance with care, use of facilities in the area, a monthly stipend, burial assistance, or a grave marker.

Thoroughly document their assets and their debt:

- Pensions
- Social Security income
- Real estate
- Bank accounts
- CDs
- Saving accounts
- Saving bonds
- Stocks
- Mutual funds
- Annuities
- Loans
- Mortgages
- Home Equity Loans
- Car Loans
- Credit Card balances

For all of the above, include account numbers, contact names, addresses, and phone numbers. I suggest listing them in an Excel spreadsheet.

Locate and place these in a safe place:

- Key(s) to Safety Deposit Box(es) at bank
- Social Security # (Get copies of these cards.)
- Medicare # (Get copies of these cards.)
- Credit cards (Get a copy of front and back of all cards along with their limits.)

- Lawyer name, firm, address, and phone number
- Tax Preparer name, firm, address, and phone number

Locate and place these in a safety deposit box:

- Birth certificates
- Wills, Living Wills, and Powers of Attorney
- House and Property Deeds
- Property Tax Bills (previous year and current year)
- Stocks
- Cemetery Lot Deeds
- Loans
- Mortgages
- All types of insurance: long-term care, life, term, medical, prescription, accident, house, car, umbrella, etc.

Depending on their trust in banks, use your organizational skills to search their home for the information you need. This might be found in their incoming mail, desk, secretary, office area, closets, cedar chests, dressers, shoe boxes, coffee cans, mini-safes, large safes, basements, safety deposit box, fire safe, etc.

Schedule a meeting with the bank customer service representative. You want them to know you personally in case you need help over the phone in the future. It reduces the risk of fraud if they know you personally.

Be aware that sometimes people try to swindle elderly people out of their money, so you want banks and companies to have tight controls on the names and beneficiaries of assets. Ensure they know you personally, and the proper precautions are in place. (*See* **Swindlers.**)

Ensure your name is listed on their bank accounts and all assets. This will require a signature by your parents. They might resist, but explain to your parents you do not want the State to get their money when they die.

Set up online access to their bank account. This is extremely important if you live 1,000 miles away as I do. You can transfer funds when it suits you. Since my name was on Mom's bank account, I met with the personal banker who provided me online access. This has been an amazing help! Mom does not know I have it or even know what it means.

Review their online bank statements and credit card bills monthly.

Add your name to their credit card accounts; then reduce their credit limit. Mom's credit card had a $13,000 limit, and she was keeping the card with her in the assisted living. She sometimes used the card to pay her drug bill or buy some things for herself. I determined that $1,000 should be the maximum limit on the card. She would not want it reduced. I had to send in my Power of Attorney to their legal department; it took two months and four phone calls to get me approved. Then I reduced her card's limit to $1,000. That gave me flexibility if we needed to use her card for her medicine or an emergency but significantly reduced the risk of fraud or theft.

Schedule meetings with contact persons for stocks, mutual funds, and annuities, so you know them personally. The good ones will request annual meetings with you to address income needs, the market, level of risk, etc. You should always include your parents if they are physically and mentally able. I stopped taking Mom when I could not perform the car-to-wheelchair transfer by myself.

If one parent has died, have extra death certificates or know how to get them (via the funeral home or the state office).

If your parents do not have a safety deposit box, get one or at least buy a fire proof metal box as a central repository for storing the important documents.

Have your name on the access list for the safety deposit box. List all their assets in this box, and you keep a copy of the list.

Locate the safety deposit keys and keep them in a safe place. You should keep one of the keys.

As a test, access the safety deposit box without your parents.

Locate property tax records and put them in the safety deposit box.

Find all insurance policies and put these in the safety deposit box. Include long-term, life, term, house, car, umbrella, etc. You do not want to miss life insurance policies or assets and leave them unclaimed.

My bachelor uncle died, and we had very limited financial data on him. He did not have a will or a checking account. I pursued the several stubs for insurance policies, and two were valid, but I wondered if I missed any. The internet and the Missouri Department of Insurance were helpful in finding the current names after some insurance companies had been sold or merged. I initiated calls to these companies, and some required specific forms to be completed for searching archived records and claiming policies.

If they have long-term care insurance, read the policy. Understand when and under what conditions payments begin.

Locate the deeds or titles for all properties and associated documents and put them in the safety deposit box. These include stocks, annuities, mutual funds, CDs, savings bonds, house deeds, and car titles.

When your parents are no longer able, who is going to handle paying the monthly bills, medical paperwork, the property taxes, and income taxes?

If you have siblings, you need to decide who will handle what specific duties. If someone is stronger in finances or lives locally, they might be the right person. In your parents' wills who is named the Executor of the Estate? This person should be involved in the decisions now.

Update the beneficiary information on all their assets. Put copies in the safety deposit box.

Locate their past federal and state income tax records.

Note on your calendar when their property taxes are due.

Get your parents' lawyer and tax preparer's names, addresses, and phone numbers.

***Critical: Ensure each parent has a Power of Attorney, will, and living will. Get **two** original signed powers of attorney for each parent because you copy it often. Your name and an alternate name should be included in the Power of Attorney.

Schedule a meeting with your parents' lawyer, if necessary, regarding names on assets, transfer at death or survivorship, estate planning, trusts, wills, powers of attorney, living wills, and beneficiaries. You want to prevent problems later and minimize inheritance taxes.

Put the original signed and notarized Powers of Attorney, wills, and living wills in the safety deposit box.

The Power of Attorney gives you the authority to handle their business while they are alive.

The assigned Executor from their wills handles their business after their death.

Ensure your parents have a living will to clarify their wishes as the end draws near.

Give a copy of the living will (legal health care directive) to the facility and to the family doctor.

Your parents will probably fight all of this because they do not want you interfering or meddling in their business. They don't want to think about death. Mom always thought of me as a child, so it was difficult for her to allow me to handle her business.

Mom's lawyer did an excellent job of preparing all the necessary documents and modifying her car title and house deed. I was so excited when I found the signed Power of Attorney in her safety deposit box that was created while Daddy was still alive giving him and me Power of Attorney (POA) for Mom. Finding this POA was like finding gold! She does not realize that I have it. Without it, I would not have been able to find out her health status remotely when she was in the hospital with an infected foot. The new Privacy Laws severely restrict what information hospitals provide. This Power of Attorney has been so valuable!

Mom has difficulty with fine motor skills, has trouble signing her name, and cannot read documents due to her macular degeneration. It was imperative that I have the Power of Attorney to take over bill paying and management of her affairs. When I started handling her business and changing her mailing address to mine, I had to fax or mail the POA to every company. With some businesses I had to work with their legal department, and it took weeks and even months to get this approved. When I changed Mom's mailing address to mine, I told the companies that Mom still resided in Missouri for tax purposes and pharmacy reasons.

Sign your name on your parents' documents and follow it with **"POA"** for Power of Attorney.

Make many extra copies of the Power of Attorney to fax or mail to all companies to change their mailing address to yours and to allow those companies to talk to you in addition to your parents.

Tip: If there is an embossed or raised seal on the Power of Attorney, lay a pencil on its side and lightly rub the lead across the seal. This will make the seal stand out, so it shows on a copy or a fax.

Schedule a meeting with the tax preparer for their annual federal and state tax returns. For tax purposes:

- File your parents' federal and state income taxes each year, including for the year they die. Even if you think you do not need to file, it is better to close out everything while you have the information than be audited several years in the future for not having filed.

- Provide the tax preparer with your parents' care facility costs.

- Provide your parents' tax preparer with all medical expenses.

- Provide your parents' tax preparer with all long-term care insurance payments.

- Draft a letter to the IRS for their doctor's signature stating your parents are unable to live independently, giving valid reasons, and need assisted living, which was definitely true for Mom. Take the letter to their family doctor for signature. Include a copy to your parents' tax preparer each year. Keep the original for future usage.

- Keep detailed records regarding the sale of your parents' furniture and belongings.

- Document the original cost of their house and any improvements.

Lost Money

Check these websites for both of your parents' names for potential unclaimed or lost money. Some States' Attorneys General also provide this information free.

- www.missingmoney.com

- www.unclaimed.org

Check this website for saving bonds: www.treasurydirect.gov

3

Your Finances

Will your parents outlive their money? If so, you, your spouse, and your siblings might need to contribute to their living expenses. If that is the case, check on Medicare and Medicaid. (*See* **Help for Elders**.)

If your parents have not adequately prepared financially for the later, expensive stages of life and do not have long-term care insurance, you will need to check on Medicare and Medicaid assistance. Some facilities will not accept Medicaid. There is a risk that you will need to assist with these expenses. That is why understanding your parents' financial status is so important. You also need to have these difficult financial discussions with your spouse and siblings as you also plan for your own retirement. You might be helping your children with college expenses or a down payment on a house. Your children might have moved back into your home after a job loss or divorce. You might experience the sandwich generation where we are **caring and paying** for our parents, ourselves, and our young, adult children. This might impact your own retirement date. It might necessitate your working several years longer.

Add money in your budget for more trips to visit your parents each year if they live in another town. My multiple trips to Missouri to see and check on Mom add over $2,500 per year to my annual expenses.

I made a choice to not work outside the home for the past five and a half years and have given up significant income. I spent two weeks there while her house was being painted. I was there another time when her roof needed repairs. I made numerous trips to clean out Mom's house. After I had the three-day auction of household goods, I felt a tremendous weight off my shoulders. Then I also helped my cousins clean out our Grandma's house, so her house and belongings could be sold. I moved items I wanted to keep to my house and need to organize them. When I get calls about Mom's house, I send out information packages and also have open houses when I am in town; I hope her house sells soon. The work is not done.

Money can impact family relationships. Even if you have a good relationship with your siblings, choices concerning money can change things. There can be arguments over who gets the parents' prized possessions. Siblings and their spouses might not think the same way you do. They might not want to spend the parents' money the way you think it should be spent. Be true to your own values for what is important.

To give me a sense of accomplishment during this time I compiled Daddy's World War II letters to Mom into a published book and wrote this.

Initially I did not know how long this period of caregiving would last. Mom's father died at 87 and her mother at 94. Mom's older brother died two years ago at 92, and her younger brother at almost 89 is in good health in an assisted living. To be honest, I did not expect Mom to live in care facilities for six and a half years. I thought her diabetes would shorten her life, but, in reality, her body organs are strong. I still don't know how long she will live. For almost sixteen years since my father died, I have been assisting Mom, taking care of her house, and providing for her needs. It has not been full-time, but it is time consuming.

There is a feeling of uncertainty or limbo. Now I need to review my choice to not work outside the home. I miss working with people, getting a sense of accomplishment, helping others, and getting paid. I have an income, but it would be beneficial to supplement that in planning for retirement. Recently I applied for several jobs with no job offer, but it could be managers are unwilling to risk hiring someone who has not worked outside the home for five and a half years. If I commit to a full-time job, will I be able to leave when her house sells? Will I be able to go there for several months if she gets ill or her health declines? Every time the phone rings at odd hours I wonder if the nurse is calling about Mom. I am uncertain about when I might need to go. I visit her three to four times per year and stay at least seven to ten days. Would I be able to get that much time off? Would it be fair to my employer? Would I be able to focus on my job? Mom wants me there all the time. I had made the decision to not move back to Mom's town, although I was there over four months the year I had her auction. Should I move her here to reduce my time out of town? When I leave, will I ever see her again? This is a difficult dilemma that I have not resolved.

I usually wait until two weeks before each trip home to book my airline ticket in case there is a change in Mom's health, and I need to drive. I drive if I stay an extended period of time to avoid extreme car rental fees. With high gas prices, it is cheaper to fly if I stay ten days or less. Flying is my default choice because it takes four days for me to drive the 2,000 miles round-trip by myself.

4

Swindlers

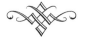

***Critical: Before bringing help into their home, put all their valuables in a safety deposit box or move the valuables to your home.**

Do not take valuables to an assisted living/skilled care facility.

Monitor their checking accounts and credit card bills monthly.

Reduce their credit card limits to $1,000 or less to minimize fraud risk.

Remove their checkbooks, credit cards, and cash when their mental capacities decline.

File a police report if anything is stolen.

Put their phone number on the National Do Not Call Registry: www.donotcall.gov

For in-home caregivers:

> » Run background checks.

> » Ask for references and call them.

I always thought that everyone is honest and trustworthy.

Unfortunately, that is not the case, so you must take precautions to prevent trouble and loss of valuables or money. You also do not want to tempt the caregivers with valuables. Once items are stolen, it is difficult to prove and nearly impossible to get them back.

There was a nice, friendly woman who worked at Mom's assisted living. She offered to take Mom out to lunch, and Mom thoroughly enjoyed the attention and the chance to go out for a meal. I did not mind that Mom paid for both of their lunches. I could see the charge on Mom's credit card or the written check. She would even take Mom shopping at J. C. Penney's, tell Mom the clothes looked nice on her, and suggest Mom buy them. That was fine; the amount of money charged was reasonable, and it gave Mom pleasure. Then I saw one charge for over $400. When I asked Mom, she said this woman picked out clothes for Mom and selected items for herself, too. The woman expected Mom to pay for everything. I told Mom she did not have to pay for the woman's items and suggested she refuse in the future. I did not alert the facility. When it happened a second time, I knew I had to take action. The woman's husband also worked at the facility, so I approached him. I explained the situation had to stop. His wife had told him Mom volunteered to buy the clothes. I told him the two amounts of almost $1,000, and he was shocked. He knew if I told the facility that one or both of them would be fired. They had three sons and needed the income. After I confronted the husband, it never happened again. Unfortunately, the woman stopped taking Mom to lunch, so Mom was the loser in several ways. I was able to return some of the clothes with the tags that did not fit or look good on Mom. I don't know if I handled it the best way, but the scam stopped.

I was using the online banking access to monitor the checks that were written by the office staff for Mom to sign to pay her bills. I noticed she was not paying some bills on time and paying other bills twice. Mom was getting too forgetful to handle this, so it was time for me to start paying Mom's bills at age 88. I discreetly took Mom's credit card and her checkbook. I informed the office of the change. When

Mom realized she did not have any money, it made her very angry, but I did not want Mom writing checks to the wrong people or someone stealing checks and emptying her bank account. I told Mom I could write checks for anything she needed. Prior to this, she would go to Walmart on the bus Wednesday afternoons and buy herself a trinket or some snacks with her charge card. Realistically, she probably should not go on the bus without supervision since she was visually impaired, could not read price tags, or see amounts charged.

When Mom was 88, it was not a good idea to leave money in her purse. I left $5 or $10 for my uncle several times, and he would say someone asked for his money. Once dementia begins and the judgment portion of their brain does not work properly, remove the credit cards, checkbooks, and cash. You feel guilty taking their cash away, but it will not be used for their benefit. Mom has a trust fund at her current facility where I keep at most $60, so if they go out to eat or bring in food, Mom can participate. The facility includes this trust fund balance with her bill and documents how any funds are spent.

When you hire an in-home caregiver, it is difficult to protect against crooks. I suggest you run a background check for a criminal record. Even if you find none, the person might be using an alias. A caregiver whom a friend's parent hired went by one name. She asked the father to make checks out to a person with a different first name, whom she said was her mother. The father was puzzled but did as she asked.

Be alert to anything that does not seem right. When the mother died, there were questions whether the caregiver caused or contributed to the mother's death. There was no proof. The father just kept saying his wife was pointing to her chest when they put her to bed; she was dead the next morning. Initially the caregiver did a good job but was not so good toward the end. My friend feels as if he should have recognized something was not right, but he thought his father was there and would handle any problems. In retrospect, the father was worse off mentally than the son realized.

His sister took their mother's engagement ring, which their dad gave her at the mother's funeral, to a jeweler for an appraisal. Their dad told her it was worth $5,000 to $10,000. The appraiser said it was worthless costume jewelry! They suspected that the in-home care provider substituted it for the real ring. Once she completed the switch, it appears she had no need for the patient, or potential witness, anymore.

Watch out for your parents "loaning" the caregiver money.

One friend said someone called him saying his grandmother owed $1,500 for Avon products!

Another friend said when she left cash in her father's wallet at the care facility, it disappeared overnight, so she stopped doing that.

Mom said some charity called on the phone, and she agreed to donate $35.

I picked up a significant check for my uncle's portion of Grandma's house sale and was having him sign it, so I could deposit it in his bank. The woman at his assisted living quickly called his daughter to find out who I was. My cousin knew about the transaction, talked to me on the phone, and told the lady I was his niece and was okay to help with the finances. She did the right thing to question who I was!

Several pairs of sterling silver earrings and fake diamond rings have disappeared; two nice afghans were missing.

This year two friends had their social security numbers compromised. People fraudulently filed tax returns using my friends' social security numbers to steal their tax refunds.

Beware of people who prey on the elderly! Keep your guard up! Minimize the ways people can take advantage of the situation.

5

Get the Memories

Ask your questions now before your parents' memories gradually fade and are lost forever. Ask lots of questions and use a tape recorder to record their memories in their own words about:

- Family history and genealogy. Document information on names of relatives, births, deaths, and burial locations.

- Your parents' meeting.

- Your dad's (and mom's) service in the war with rank, branch, location, and assignment. Did he or she receive any medals and why?

- Your ethnic heritage and family migration.

- Any special family events and favorite stories.

- Any family heirlooms and their original owners.

- Their defining moments.

Take your parents back to where they grew up or where their parents or grandparents lived, and let them tell you stories about their youth.

I admit I was not paying close attention when Grandma kept repeating our family history. It was boring and dry. Now I wish I had taken notes on those stories! At least she was excellent at documenting the family genealogy, so we do have recorded information. She traced the family roots to a relative who fought in the Revolutionary War, so she and Mom could join Daughters of the American Revolution (DAR).

Several years ago I took Mom and her brother to the cemetery where her grandparents were buried. That visit encouraged many memories and stories, and I took pictures of the tombstones and name of the cemetery for my family records.

I also took them to the farm where my great-great-grandparents and their children lived. The current owners remembered my family name and allowed me to visit the family cemetery plot which was originally behind their home that burned. The tombstones have fallen over and are covered with grass, but that confirmed the specific location of my great-great-great-grandparents' graves.

Now Mom cannot remember much of her youth or her husband. If I mention names, she remembers who people were. But it is too late to ask about family history or events.

Here is a reverse memory suggestion. One family had a father with Alzheimer's disease. They wrote out individual memories the son and grandchildren had with their parent and grandparent and placed the pieces of paper in a jar. Each day one memory was selected from the jar and that beautiful thought brought him a moment of joy when his own memory had faded.

6

Preparing Now

Any major change, such as breaking a hip or stopping driving, could require an immediate relocation in their living quarters.

Consider moving your parents into your home or a sibling's home. Think about this now and discuss it with your spouse. You need to know your decision before the choice becomes an emergency. For me this was not an option. Mom wanted me to move into her home, so she could stay there. I would move her back to her house for my one-to two-week visits, but I knew I could not live there until her death. Our personalities were not compatible; we do things differently, and it would cause me a mental breakdown. Mom seemed to criticize whatever I did. Nothing I did seemed to suit her or was enough. I believe she did this to make me better. Regardless of the reason, it was demeaning and unhealthy for me.

If your parents moved in with you:

- Would your spouse stay?
- Would your sanity stay?
- Could you keep your job?

Only you and your spouse know the answers.

With the extreme expense of skilled care facilities, some adult children are avoiding or delaying it by modifying their homes. One person built a new home and finished the upstairs for his mother's suite with an elevator. They included an intercom system to communicate between the two floors. The mother joins the husband and wife for meals often, and it is easy to drop off groceries and check on her. Yet they have their own separate space.

Another friend added on a mother-in-law suite to his house. He figured they would more than recover the money by keeping her out of a skilled care facility for several years. In the future when the mother no longer uses the area, it would increase their home size and its value. She is still a part of their family and shares some meals with them but has her own space. They built it while the mother was in her early 70s.

You need to prepare for the stages ahead as your parents age, and their independence declines. If there are no major health issues, your parents may be able to remain in their home or current residence into their 80s and maybe 90s with minimal assistance. But if there are major health issues like dementia, diabetes, macular degeneration, impaired vision, heart problems, Alzheimer's disease, or Parkinson's disease, they might need to change living quarters much earlier.

7

Out of Town

Concern: As your parents' health deteriorates, at some point you will not be able to move them to a different town. Consider if you must move them, what is the optimal timeframe?

If your parents live in another town or out of state, you need to consider if you are going to move them to your town or the town of one of your siblings, and whether you will force a move. Forcing them to move puts incredible pressure on them, but even more on you. An only child friend insisted her mother move to her town, about eight hours away. My friend, the daughter, actually had a stroke in her 50s because of the stress of emptying the mother's house, selling the home, and moving her mother in a short period of time. The mother handled the move without any health problems but was never happy away from her hometown and friends even though she was with her daughter and grandchildren. It is a significant decision with risks to your parents and you.

Since I am an only child and live 1,000 miles away from my mother, I asked her if she wanted to move to my town where her only child and only grandchild live. Her answer was, "Why would I ever want to do that?" She had lived in her hometown all but fourteen years of her life, and during those years she always wanted to return to her hometown. She did not even consider what would be easier for me. I did not force the move since it might cause her to have a stroke or possibly me to have a stroke! You must think about the potential outcome before making decisions.

The other major consideration is that at some point you **will not be able** to move your parents to your town or the town where a sibling lives. So you need to weigh the pros and cons concerning making them move and if, at some point, you must force the move.

Finances should be considered although this is not the only deciding factor. Assisted living and skilled care facilities in some areas of the country, especially large cities, are more expensive than others.

Visit facilities and check prices and options in all potential locations.

My girlfriend asked me, "Have you thought again about moving your mom to your town?" After her mother had a stroke, with the doctor's assistance she moved her mother near her in a wonderful skilled care facility. Her mother had previously refused to move but seemed to accept her new surroundings.

Mom could be very angry as she was when I had the auction, or she might give up or have a seizure like she did the week before the auction. It is a very risky, difficult move, and I am not sure of the rewards. I am still thinking about it. When I asked her years ago, she emphatically did not want to leave her hometown. She might have changed her mind since few people visit her, but she cannot remember if anybody comes. She is lucky that one church friend visits her weekly. I visited her recently, and she gets spoiled with seeing me daily and my giving her much attention. Then she wants me to come back soon.

The bottom line is: Would she be willing to move or fight it? I am still considering the answer.

Is it too late to move her? Since she is incontinent, and I cannot transfer her, I would need two people to travel with me by air. She hates to fly, but there is a non-stop flight, and the doctor could provide a sedative. Again, I am still considering this.

8

End of Driving

Are you willing to ride with your parents or allow your children to ride with them?

Night vision goes first, and most seniors realize when they should stop driving at night. They also realize when to stop driving on the highways. It is very difficult to give up driving totally because it takes away their freedom and impacts their way of life.

Has their eyesight declined? If they are having trouble shuffling across the floor, do you really think they could quickly hit the car brake?

You will know when your parents need to stop driving, and you must take action to prevent them from killing themselves or killing someone else because of poor vision, judgment, or reflexes. Could you live with that on your conscience? Get the eye doctor or family doctor to be the bad guy by stating their vision or mobility is inadequate if that is the case. Write an anonymous letter to the Department of Motor Vehicles and request they have the parent take the driving test. If you ask, NC DMV will send a letter saying the parent has been "randomly selected" to be retested due to their age. Or take the keys away, or sell the car. You cannot afford to be weak about this issue. In an accident, if there is not sufficient insurance, the parent or estate can be sued, too. Fortunately, Mom realized her vision was declining and stopped driving at about 84. It was still very traumatic for her when I sold her prized Cadillac Brougham though.

After Mom stopped driving, her younger brother volunteered to take her for groceries and errands once a week. Also, she started Meals on Wheels to supplement her food supply because she was cooking less. This enabled her to stay in her home for a couple more years. She already had a good yard man to take care of the outside. This meant she was spending more time alone since she was not able to go out with her friends. A church member picked her up on Sundays to attend church for several years. She gradually was having more trouble getting in and out of their vehicle, so they declined to continue. She had attended church her whole life; that was really hard on her, but I understood it from a liability perspective.

When your parents stop driving, they need someone to get their groceries, run errands, and take them to doctors' appointments. This is also the time to start evaluating their next move to different housing or a facility.

Several years later I could tell my uncle's vision had declined, and he should not be driving. I discussed this with my cousins, who did not want to confront him. I set up an appointment with the eye doctor, and my uncle went with me nervously. Fortunately, he just needed one cataract lens cleaned with a minor surgical procedure. I took him back for his recheck after the procedure, and he got the green light to legally drive. It was a happy story! He continued safely driving short distances for several years then stopped driving when a heart issue required him to move into assisted living.

Get your parents' legal state photo identification cards at the state motor vehicle bureau when they stop driving. This is needed for personal identification as a replacement for the driver's license. If a driver's license has expired, it is not considered a valid ID. They might need photo identifications at some time.

9

Transition Period

Keep your parents in their current living quarters as long as possible because the cost jumps exponentially when they move to an assisted living and then to a skilled care facility (nursing home).

Your parents are probably living in their own home, but as they age or have more health issues, you need to consider making some modifications to reduce the risks of accidents.

- Add grab bars or handrails to ease entering and exiting the tub or shower. The major concern of injury in the home is the bathtub or shower, so reduce this risk. Realize they might not bathe often for fear of falling.

- Keep your parents walking and mobile as long as possible.

- Remove throw rugs and other tripping hazards. Your goal is to avoid their breaking hips, which increase the risk of death.

- Move furniture to open walkways.

- Buy canes and/or walkers, as needed. Some walkers have seats and brakes. Do not let pride or ego get in their way of using an aid if they need it. Say you want them to avoid broken hips; someone they know will have had a broken hip, so this works. The plastic skis or ends on the walkers wear out, so check them periodically. Some people use tennis balls on the walker feet, but these do not work well on carpeting.

- Get them Life Alert-type buttons; encourage them to wear them. These systems easily connect through the home phone line. The alerts can be worn around the neck or on the wrist. You will know when it is time to get them one. I got Mom's when she was about 80 and living alone. The cost (about $30 per month) is worth the comfort of knowing a parent who falls can get immediate help. Plus, it is much cheaper than assisted living. This provides you some peace of mind.

- Order Meals on Wheels to be delivered during the week. As long as they are still driving, they can get groceries and cook. Watch their refrigerator for spoiled food or signs they are not buying groceries or not eating well. Watch for loss of weight or muscle tone. I could tell my uncle was losing weight and muscle tone, plus his refrigerator did not have much food when I checked. So I suggested to my cousins that he needed Meals on Wheels. They did not want to get into an argument with him, so I told them I would be the "bad guy." I ordered Meals on Wheels to start the next Monday. I called my uncle and told him that I started them, and he said, "Okay." I asked if he wanted me to pay for the first month, and he replied that he could handle the payments. Having Meals on Wheels delivered ensures someone checks on them five days a week, and they eat one nutritious meal per day at a small cost. Just as importantly, it gives them some social contact. You can pay weekly or monthly.

- Consider if a wheelchair ramp could be added to their house, if needed.

- Consider installing a stair lift to carry them upstairs. It costs several thousand dollars, but if they are mentally sharp, this could delay their moving to a facility and save money.

- Consider buying a van with a wheelchair lift for the other parent to drive. This will extend their independence. You can have hand controls installed if their reflexes are good.

Concerns while they live independently are:

- Fire from a stove burner being left on
- Adequate nutrition with less cooking
- Medicines on time
- Showering alone with the risk of falling
- Blood sugar fluctuations for diabetics
- Reduced vision from macular degeneration, cataracts, or glaucoma
- Bills getting paid on time

  Try to set up draft payments, so bills will be paid regularly.

Remove valuables from the home before bringing in help. (*See* **Swindlers**.)

Initially consider getting them one or more persons to:

- Clean the house or apartment.
- Do yard work.
- Pick up groceries and medicines if they are not driving.
- Prepare some or all meals.
- Shower and dress them.

Have them enjoy whatever brings them happiness before they move into an assisted living or a skilled care facility.

10

Preventing Falls

Put safety first. Broken hips significantly increase their risk of death. You need to take precautions to avoid falls. Follow the steps mentioned above.

For many years during my visits when Mom lived in the assisted living, I would move her back into her home. She fell three times while in my care. She could not get up on her own, and I could not lift her weight. On those occasions I called EMTs, who were extremely kind and helpful. She did not break anything and did not go to the hospital. Luckily, there was no charge if they do not take the person to the hospital! They knew she was in an assisted living when I was not in town. She enjoyed being in her home when she could, so the reward was worth the risk. It was embarrassing to me, but I had few options since she weighs 160 pounds.

One time Mom's ceiling leaked, and her large Oriental rug got wet. I pulled it outside to dry. Later I told Mom to stand back because I was pulling it back into the house. Once I got the large, heavy roll started, I wanted to keep going. She had to watch my every move and was too close; I bumped her with the rug, and she went down like a slow falling bowling pin. There she was, sprawled over the rug, and crying out, "I can't breathe!" I replied, "If you can talk, you can breathe!" I had to laugh to keep from crying. I got a stool and pillow to put under her chest until EMT could get there to pick her up, again!

I asked Mom to try driving her friend's motorized wheelchair. Then I suggested she try driving the one at Walmart, but she would not touch them. Maybe with her vision impairment and lack of depth perception, she could not see well enough. Also, there was an incident at her meal table at the assisted living when one woman's wheelchair hit the table, knocked it into Mom, and bruised her arm and leg. I guess she felt they could be dangerous.

I signed a form that allows the skilled care facility to keep two bedrails on Mom's bed. Since she is not mobile at all and does not remember that, I do not want her getting out of bed without someone there.

Keep your parents up and moving! Mom was in the hospital for a bleeding ulcer for eight days while I had the auction of her belongings. I do not know if the blood transfusions contributed to the loss of her ability to walk, but I do know that loss of muscle tone in the legs played a key role. One time I was on crutches for three weeks, and my leg muscles atrophied quickly. I requested the doctor prescribe Mom physical therapy, which he did. She took the therapy for some months but complained it was too painful and gave up. At 90 she did not have the determination to walk again.

When Mom could no longer walk and started using a wheelchair, she would not even try pushing the wheels to get where she wanted. She tried a few times but either was not strong enough or not motivated. I thought being in a wheelchair would bother Mom. Someone pushes her to meals, church, and bingo. She seems fine telling someone else to do things for her and being waited on like a princess. People are so different. I would not want to be pushed and would insist on doing it myself!

The wheelchair brings with it all kinds of complications: loss of muscle tone, urinary tract infections, bedsores or boils, incontinence, and weight gain. Sometimes it can lead to depression when people are unable to go out of their facility.

Now that Mom is in a wheelchair she might as well be in prison. Her quality of life has declined significantly. One person cannot transfer her, so I am not able to take her out to eat, shop, concerts, or travel — her favorite things. The aides at the facility did load her in my rental car, I drove her to her brother's assisted living, he came out to see her for a few minutes, and then I drove her around town, by her house and her mother's house, etc. Then the aides got her out of the car. Mom still loves to go places, so once in a while they take Mom and other residences in the special van out to eat or on a ride.

11

Home Design

Concerns:

- Are their bedroom and bath on the main floor?

- Are there stairs to get into the home?

- Can you adapt the house for wheelchair accessibility?

- Are the halls and doors wide enough for walkers or wheelchairs?

- Can a stackable washer/dryer be installed on the main floor?

- Is it close to a grocery store?

- Is it close to a pharmacy?

- Is their home on a bus line, or is there convenient transportation?

- Is there public transportation for seniors, like OATS buses in Missouri?

12

Plan for the Next Phase

Issues:

- What is the right choice for your parents?
- What is the right choice for you?
- What are you willing to sacrifice for your parents?
- What will your spouse tolerate?
- How much will your siblings help?
- Are your parents safe?
- Is it time to move them where they are safe?
- Are your parents willing to leave their hometown?
- Are you going to force the move?
- Are there excellent facilities in the current hometown?
- Is there a hospital in their current hometown?
- What is the difference in costs between their hometown and yours?
- Will you ask your parents to live with you initially?

If your parents are still in their own home, hopefully you have already decided whether your parents can move in with you or one of your siblings. You and your spouse must have discussed this serious question. Are your parents difficult or demanding? Are yours and your parents' temperaments compatible? No matter how loving you are, it is still difficult having different generations living together.

My childhood summer sitter had her elderly mother living with her family in an upstairs bedroom. This woman had amazing patience in dealing with me and her two daughters, but the elderly mother upset her daughter at everything she did. Sometimes the daughter would scream at her mother for messing up her kitchen. Usually the mother stayed upstairs out of the way; I felt sorry for both of them. It was not healthy for either one.

Ask where your parents would like to live when they leave their home. Some of their friends will have already made this move. Do not be surprised if they ask to live with you! They might want you, especially if you are single, to move into their house with them! You must have considered these options and made a decision before they ask. Of course, they probably will not want to leave their home voluntarily.

Some parents are wise enough to know they should never live with their children; it is too much to ask and not healthy for all involved. They refuse, even if the offer is made.

Delay moving your parents out of their home as long as possible but put their safety as the most critical factor in your decision. You do not want them leaving doors unlocked, letting in strangers, falling on the stairs, going hungry, or eating spoiled food. Usually when their memory is affected, their judgment is impaired as well.

If your parents are living with a sibling or you, you do not want you or your sibling to be injured in trying to move or help your parents. You do not want you or your sibling to become mentally frazzled. Hopefully, you will realize when it is time to move them. They might not agree. Being a care provider can be draining, even from a distance.

Required roles:

- Caregiver/Advocate, even if they are in a facility
- Financial person to handle bills, insurance, taxes, etc.
- Driver for errands
- Driver and second set of ears for doctors' visits
- Planner to move your parents
- Person to downsize and disperse belongings (sorting, sale, etc.)
- Seller of their house

These roles can be divided or shared among the siblings depending on the circumstances. These roles might change through the years. It is overwhelming and exhausting for one person to handle it all. Even if you are not a full-time caregiver, it takes a significant amount of time, and working from another town makes it even harder. For almost sixteen years I have maintained Mom's house, prepared all papers for taxes, sent gifts and cards, bought her clothes, managed her medical and prescription insurance, and checked on medicines, doctor visits, etc. For six and a half years I have interfaced with the facility on her condition and needs. For three years I have handled Mom's checking account, bills, house, assets, insurance, etc. It seems like something needs to be done every day, whether it is paying the yardman, filing a piece of mail, or talking to the nurses at the facility. It means doing work that is not fun. Plus I try to talk to Mom daily.

Many men just do not understand what is involved in caring for aging parents, so if you have brothers or husbands, do not expect much cooperation, contribution, or willingness to help from them. Sympathy, empathy, caring, listening, and helping are usually not their strengths. They do not understand that clothes, jewelry, hair, and nails are important to a woman. Do not be upset if your brothers or husbands are clueless, and do not seem to care like you do. Their standards of care are probably not the same as yours. Do not expect their help. There are some exceptions. Be pleasantly surprised if they offer and then do it. Consider this when deciding where your parents should live and who is going to be the primary care provider.

If one spouse has dementia or Alzheimer's disease, you may need to move this partner to a special care facility for the **safety of the well partner**. This is difficult and sad. One friend had to move her stepmother into a special memory unit but put her dad in an assisted living. He was sharp enough to understand the need for this although it was still difficult emotionally.

What is the outcome you desire in moving them? You want it to be a safe place that is the best choice for them and you. You want your parents in a beautiful surrounding with tasty, nutritious food and caring, pleasant aides and nurses. The bottom line: Would you want to live there?

Mom developed macular degeneration and became visually im-paired, which she tried to hide or deny. This raised a red flag about her using the stove to cook and possibly starting a fire. Also, I did not want her eating spoiled food without realizing it or letting strangers into her home. At times you will need to be a detective to understand the real situation. Your parents will try to hide their declining conditions from you.

Mom insisted on sleeping upstairs although there is a bedroom and full bath on the main floor. I suggested Mom sleep downstairs, but she refused. It was scary watching her climb up and down the stairs. Sometimes she got stuck on the stairway and wanted me to help her. I was afraid she would make both of us fall. This was another warning sign she needed to move.

Mom also showed signs of something I identified as "Sundowner's Syndrome." When the sun went down, she became very fearful and paranoid and locked herself in her upstairs bedroom. In the winter that meant she would carry a tray of food upstairs for supper. When I was visiting her, she told me she saw a man watching her house. It was just a shadow, but it seemed real to her. She called the police literally over fifty times in one year because she thought someone was trying to break into her home although there was never any evidence of a break-in attempt. The police were wasting their manpower, so, understandably, they requested the Division of Aging have someone evaluate Mom. She passed the test just fine during the day! I did not want outsiders to decide Mom's fate, so I knew it was time for her to move to an assisted living at least to save the police officers' sanity! Mom refused to leave.

It was obvious to me she needed to move to a facility, but she would not discuss it, consider it, and was unwilling to go. Her attitude was that she was in charge, and it was none of my business. I seemed powerless to force it to happen unless I pursued Guardianship, a legal designation which can be costly and difficult to prove it is necessary. Periodically I sent letters to her doctor to document her behavior changes, like the police calls, fear at night, vision of lights on the ceiling, etc.

When her Meals on Wheels lunch was late one day, her blood sugar imbalance caused her to fall. Her yard man found her quickly, but she cut her scalp and required numerous stitches in her head and a brief hospital stay. Because I had kept the doctor informed of her increasing dementia, he put her in an assisted living to recover from the injury but told me he could only keep her there three weeks. I told him that was enough time for her to realize she should be there. Since it was winter, she stayed a few weeks longer. It was a gradual acceptance; she was no longer lonesome! By that time she realized she liked having people around, and it was great having someone cook, wash dishes, clean her room, and do her laundry. She stayed by her own choice. The doctor was wonderful in helping get her where she needed to be.

Because she was unwilling to sleep on the first floor, and she fell several times that required EMT to pick her up, on my visits I could no longer bring her back to her home at age 89. She was very angry that I would not take her home. That was hard on both of us, but it was the right decision for our safety. She could no longer enjoy her beautiful belongings.

Investigate options now before an emergency forces an urgent change.

Per www.wikipedia.com: "A study by the U.S. Department of Health and Human Services says that four out of every ten people who reach age 65 will enter a nursing home at some point in their lives. About 10 percent of the people who enter a nursing home will stay there five years or more."

- Investigate available housing options in your parents' town and your current town.
- Ask your friends what facilities have worked well for their parents.
- Ask your parents' friends what facilities have worked for them.
- Check on apartments for the elderly with one or two meals provided per day.
- Check on assisted living and their services.
- Check on skilled care facilities.
- Will your parents get any Medicare or Medicaid assistance?

If your parents are in the hospital, the social worker will assist you in getting the appropriate facility space fast.

Ask the family doctor which facilities he or she visits and recommends. Mom did not want to change doctors, so this was a limiting factor.

Visit potential facilities. Here are some questions:

- Is the location convenient for you and your siblings?
- What is the basic cost and what does that include?
- What are additional options and their costs?
- What is the cost for a private room?
- If the spouse moves into the same room, what is the additional charge?

- Is there an upfront buy-in fee? Is this ever reimbursed?
- Do they accept Medicare and Medicaid?
- Do they have openings?
- Is there a waiting list?
- Is there a fee to be added to the waiting list?
- How many meals are served each day?
- Does each room have a private bathroom?
- Is the bathroom wheelchair accessible?
- Is housekeeping and laundry included?
- Does the facility have call lights or bells?
- What is the target response time?
- Is transportation provided?
- For what services can transportation be used?
- Is there an extra charge for transportation?
- Can people in wheelchairs be transported?
- How often do doctors visit?
- What type of doctors visit?
- Does a podiatrist visit?
- Is physical therapy available at the facility?
- Are haircuts and shampoos available in-house?
- Is there an extra charge?
- Can a woman have a manicure?
- Is the facility clean and pleasant?
- Does the facility have a bad odor?
- Ask to see the Activities Sheet.
- Is there a weekly religious service?

- Are aides helpful and pleasant, or do they look overworked?
- Is TV cable available? Is it an extra fee?
- Observe the dining hall during meal time or have a meal at the facility.
- Observe other residents' alertness, grooming, and level of care.

Costs go up exponentially with additional care. Only move to the level care required at this immediate time.

Some facilities will not accept Medicare or Medicaid clients. That is why it is important to know your parents' finances before you move them into a facility and know if they will get any financial assistance. Check for details on the websites listed in **Help for Elders**. Medicaid provides assistance for people with limited assets. Medicare pays for short stays in facilities after a hospital stay for a serious illness and also covers portions of other medical expenses.

Good skilled care facilities have waiting lists. If your parents are currently in an assisted living, you should investigate the next level of care, decide on one, and add their names with your phone number to the waiting list. Some places require a deposit to be added to the waiting list. Understand how their waiting list works. If your parent moves to the top of the list, yet you are not ready to move them, do they drop your parent off the list?

I got the list of the two skilled care facilities that Mom's family doctor visited monthly. I moved Mom from the hospital into the one that had an opening, and I had her name added to the waiting list at the other one. An opening was available at the second one in a month. Sadly, someone had to die for an opening to occur, and Mom knew the woman! At that time I was not satisfied with the first facility's response time and the bathroom situation, so I moved her to the other facility. It was not my plan to move her after one month; I did give the facility a chance to prove itself. In fact, one of Mom's best friends was at this first facility, and I enjoyed seeing her. I just wanted to keep all my options available. As it turned out, the food was better at the first place!

Here are some options to consider:

- How much can you help?
- Do you work outside the home?
- How flexible are your working hours?
- How much **will** your siblings help?
- Bring part-time help into the home for meals, bathing, and dressing (probably during the day.)
- Take them to Senior Day Care. (*See* **Help for Elders.**)
- Bring full-time aides into the home.

One friend has two caregivers. Each one stays in the home for 24 hours per day for 7 days and alternates weeks with the other person. This has enabled my friend to stay in her home which was built for wheelchair accessibility. My friend is still able to transfer to her wheelchair with only one person's help.

The following choices mean your parents' belongings need to be downsized.

- If a parent lives in a location far away from their children, consider moving them close to a child.
- Is it time to move the parents in with a child or for a child to move in with the parents?
- Move them to an apartment/condo (no yard, less space to maintain, and if not one floor, with an elevator and no steps).
- Move them to an apartment/condo on one floor or with an elevator in a retirement center with one or two meals daily (with optional care like bathing, dispensing medicine, etc.).

Mom's friend moved into a senior independent living apartment complex with two meals (breakfast and lunch) provided daily and has successfully lived there for six years. The food is wonderful.

The elderly people play bridge and are still active and vital. A van is provided for errands and doctors' appointments. Mom could not move there because she needed three meals per day with her diabetes and impaired vision.

- Move them to an assisted living with optional care level packages.

    This is usually one room with a bathroom and three meals per day. Some facilities add on charges for: adult diapers, laundry, dispensing medicine, hair care, bathing/dressing, transportation, etc. Fortunately, Mom's assisted living had one set price and did not have add-on options. Sometimes people cannot stay in an assisted living if they are in wheelchairs or are incontinent.

- Move them to a skilled care facility (nursing home).

For assisted living and skilled care facility:

- Ask what their target response time is.
- Eat a meal at the facility or at least visit during meal time. See what is served and how much food is left on the plates.

Assisted living and skilled care facilities will do assessments on what services are required by your parents at this time. This will help determine where they need to move.

13

Selecting Skilled Care Facility
(Nursing Home)

Family Doctor Visits

Find out which facilities your parents' family doctor visits.
This was my primary factor in selecting Mom's facility. I checked with
Mom's family doctor to see which facilities he visits monthly; then I
selected one of those two. She did not want to change doctors, and it
made things much simpler for him to visit her.

The podiatrist visits every other month to cut toenails.

Costs

Mom's rate in a small Midwest town just increased to $157/day.
There are no add-on costs at her facility. The price of facilities in major
cities is more expensive. This should be considered when deciding to
move the parent but should not be the only factor.

The beauty of Mom's skilled care facility is that everything but
cable is included in the base price. That includes adult diapers, false
teeth cleaner, showers, haircuts, shampoos, transportation to doctors'
appointments, in addition to administering medicines. There are no
hidden costs or surprises, although it is certainly not cheap.

I provide for Mom: lip balm, hand lotion, nail polish and remover, comb, Butt Paste, over the counter supplements, afghans, wheelchair cushions, and a humidifier.

Private Room

Mom could afford a private room, and I knew she would prefer having her things in her own room.

Bathroom

I initially had Mom in a skilled care facility with a shared bathroom between two rooms. The bathroom was not large enough to be wheelchair accessible, with two people for the transfer. Also, I did not want her to share a bathroom. Her friend at the same facility had issues with being locked out of her bathroom, and Mom did not need that drama. I was not satisfied with the responsiveness at the first place, so I moved her to another facility when it became available. As it turned out, the food was better at the first place, but the responsiveness, her room, bathroom size, and facility décor were better at the second. So there are tradeoffs to consider when selecting a facility. You want the best quality of life for your parents.

Call Response Time

Push the call button and check the response time when you are visiting your parents, and they need something. If it takes ten minutes or longer, that is too long. Discuss it with the administrator.

I conducted several tests to see how long it took at the first skilled care facility for staff to respond when the call button was pushed. The call buttons lit lights located on the outside of the room and on a central monitor. On several occasions the response time was over ten minutes, which I did not consider acceptable. The director would not tell me their expected or average response time.

At the current facility, the aides have monitors on their belts that show which call buttons have been pushed. They usually respond in two or three minutes, but it might take up to ten minutes to get a second person to take Mom to the bathroom. At least they quickly check for a life threatening condition. This facility told me they measure their response time and aim for less than five minutes.

Food

The quality and quantity of food is important, but it is not the only deciding factor. My uncle loves the food at his assisted living and that is such a blessing. Mom's assisted living facility had good food for many years, but as they accepted more Medicaid patients, their food quality declined. When I asked about this, they said they had less money coming in. This was one reason I moved Mom out of the assisted living; the other reason was she needed more care since she was now in a wheelchair. Her doctor confirmed this when she was leaving the hospital and had the social worker assist me in locating a skilled care facility opening.

Food is the highlight of their day. I selected the skilled care facility with the best response time, beautiful surroundings, the best care in Mom's town, and the most expensive. I just wish the food was better. It is institutional bland food with not enough fresh fruits and vegetables. I complained in writing to the kitchen manager once about the evening meal food quality and lack of quantity; I do not consider Cheetos and potato chips as vegetables. I was not happy with the dry hamburgers and tough skin on the hot dogs. Then several months later, after checking the food, I complained to a Board Member, who knew my family. He sent a nice response, said his mother-in-law lived at the facility, and his wife visited daily. He had discussed my letter with the kitchen manager. He said dietary restrictions limited their choices. I do think the quantity of the evening meal has improved, and the skin on their hot dogs is not as tough. Mom got to be her age by eating lots of fruits and vegetables and many of them fresh. When I brought in fresh food, such as peaches, tomatoes, cantaloupe, and watermelon, from the farmers' market last summer, the people at Mom's table just loved it. (Beware that some people have food allergies; check their meal cards on the table.) I do not know what else to do to improve the taste and quality of the food. Currently Mom is having more difficulty eating (probably a vision and dexterity issue) and swallowing her food. She has been moved to a table where an aide is nearby to help. While I am there, I sit with her, cut her meat, and help her eat.

If your parents have any food allergies or dislikes, make sure the facility marks it on their meal card along with what they like to drink with meals.

You can request special food supplements. For several months Mom was drinking Ensure at one meal a day. Now they offer her yogurt after most meals. If your parents are not eating well due to poor vision, chewing/teeth issues, or swallowing problems, they might need a supplement like Ensure, Boost, or yogurt. One factor which sometimes affects the food intake of seniors is a partial loss of their senses of taste and smell which occurs as a person ages. This taste loss may result in a general loss of interest in food among older persons.

Room Location

At some point you might want to ask the facility if a room opens closer to the dining room that you want it for your parents. They make that trip six times each day. Although it is good exercise for them now, at some point they could feel overwhelmed by the distance.

Activities

Check the activities sheet. Mom really likes playing bingo, attending church, and listening to any musical entertainment. Let the people know what your parents would enjoy attending. If they have an exercise session (usually sitting in a chair and moving their arms), ensure your parents attend. Mom's facility knows she likes to go on the van.

Showers

Mom refused to take showers on many occasions. She was fearful of falling, plus the physical exertion seemed overwhelming. She would even fight the aides at the assisted living. When I gave her showers, I would get soaking wet and be drained. I told the caregivers that she did not get a choice. With her incontinent issues and diabetes, she definitely needed to be washed, plus she always felt better after she took a shower.

At the assisted living they put up a schedule on her bathroom door listing the specific two days a week she took showers. This reduced the arguments.

Transportation

- Does the facility have a van to take your parents to doctors' appointments?
- Is the van accessible for wheelchairs?

Normally I can only ask for the van to take Mom to doctors' appointments. They will not take her to get her nails polished or to the beauty shop. Her regular doctor and foot doctor come to the facility. As an exception, they did take her in the van to the book signing of her husband's World War II letters.

Bottom Line: In comparison to available facilities would you want to live here? I use the same guideline for Mom as I did selecting daycare for my child. As long as you would feel comfortable staying at the place, then your parents will, too.

Are your parents social like Mom? If so, and the people are alert, your parents will enjoy talking to them and will make new friends. Mom was so lonesome in her house by herself after she stopped driving but would not admit it. She enjoyed the people at the assisted living and had many friends, but now she is not capable of carrying on much of a conversation or remembering much of her past. Now she just sits in the lobby and watches people come and go.

Nurses/Aides at Facilities

Be an advocate for your parents.

Only escalate major issues up the chain of command.

Do not sweat the small stuff!

Do the nurses/aides like their jobs? Are they helpful and friendly?

It does not cost you anything to give the workers kind words or compliments.

There are several managers and levels of skills working at the facilities: Director, Administrator, head nurse, registered nurses, certified nursing assistants, aides, kitchen manager, kitchen staff, laundry staff, cleaning staff, maintenance, finance person, and social worker. Treat all these people with respect and kindness. You will need their help, plus you want your parents treated with respect. Take any medical issues or questions to the nurse at the main station for your parents' wing. If that person cannot resolve your issue, then go to the head nurse. The aides can answer your questions about daily behavior, clothes, or needs.

If you tell someone on first shift, do not assume the message gets communicated to second shift. Aides change patients and halls periodically, so do not assume the help is there for weeks at a time. From my observations, there seems to be a high turnover rate.

Mom's facility orders her medicine from a local pharmacy. Her facility is unwilling to do mail order, which would save Mom money. I escalated this issue to the Director, who said that was not part of their procedures. She stood firm. This facility is a non-profit and has a Board of Directors, but I have not taken this issue to them. I did take the poor food quality and quantity to the Board of Directors after I complained to the kitchen manager first and gave her a chance to respond.

I also complained boldly when Mom's two new, nice afghans were missing. I planned to buy two new ones, and I did not want them to be taken! Thankfully, they are still there.

Most of the nurses/aides at Mom's assisted living and now at her skilled care facility are very caring, patient, and kind. They seem to do this work because they like helping others. I have made surprise visits to the facility, and Mom is always well groomed. A few times her hair has been too long, but that is a minor problem. They notify me of any change, such as a urinary tract infection, a fall out of bed or her wheelchair, or a different behavior.

Nurses and aides at the care facilities have difficult jobs, so please be patient and kind with them. You do not want them to abuse your loved ones while you are not there! They care about the patients but not as much as you do. Realize that these people are probably making low wages. Their jobs are demanding emotionally to be patient and kind when they do not feel like it, or the patients are not cooperating. The patients do not intend to be difficult, but many times they are. Daily Mom demands to wear earrings, a necklace, two bracelets, and two rings. Most people in the facility do not wear jewelry other than a wedding band, but Mom does not feel dressed without her jewelry and pretty clothes. She always looks nice.

Care providers at Mom's current facility are not allowed to accept gifts. Ask at your parents' facility if there is any way you can reward the special caregivers. At Mom's assisted living I gave one great nurse some of Mom's nicer clothes when they did not fit her any more.

One surprise benefit of publishing Daddy's World War II letters to Mom as a book was that the aides would come into Mom's room to read the letters. This gave Mom more attention and care.

14

Emotional Issues for Your Parents

Feelings Are Not Wrong.

Your parents have feelings, and so do you. Their feelings are important and are not wrong. Be sensitive to them. You need to honor these feelings and consider them in making the best decision for all people involved. You do need to take action to reduce the anger and frustration for all parties.

Fear

Mom has always lived in a place of fear. Whenever she was alone, she was fearful. My aunt was wonderful to stay with Mom for several weeks after Daddy died. She gradually reduced the time she was there to help Mom through this transition.

Mom has a tape playing in her mind that says, "What if? What if something bad happens? What if something happened to her only child?" When I was four, my neighbor was watching me in a dime store, and I said I was going back to Mom. When Mom saw the neighbor, she asked the neighbor where I was, and the neighbor said she thought I was with Mom. I was only a few aisles away looking at all the pretty things, but Mom panicked. She would never let me out of her sight after that. She felt guilty that she did not protect me, but I was fine. So any time I returned home, she did not want me out of her sight.

Recognize your parents will be afraid to move into a new facility. Do what you can to ease the transition. Check for family friends on the list of residents.

Anger About Loss of Control and Freedom

Always remember there is a beautiful young person trying to get out of that old body. Your parents might take their anger out on you, but you are not the only reason for their anger. Aging and having less control over your body is difficult. If your parents are angry, they might not be specifically mad at you but at their current condition. They want things to stay the way they were forever, such as living in their house and driving their car.

They will be angry at you for making them take a bath. It is not nice, but sometimes I had to tell Mom, "You smell." They might be angry at you for making them put on clean clothes. They might be angry at you for making a doctor's appointment with the neurologist because they feel there is nothing wrong with them. They might not have the energy or feel like doing any of these things, but they need to be done.

Realize that parents are angry because:

- They are losing control of their life and choices.
- They do not like being told what to do.
- They cannot drive.
- They have lost their freedom and independence.
- Their bodies do not work well anymore.
- They do not have much energy.
- They might be in pain.
- Their friends are dead or dying.
- Their future is dim, and death is imminent.

Leaving the home they have known for decades is extremely difficult emotionally for your parents. They know they are losing control of their life, their choices, their freedom, and their future. They know it is the beginning of the end. It means they are one step closer to the grave. Some will leave willingly, but others will fight you and refuse. There will be tears for your parents and you at these major transitions.

They realize they will no longer be able to go out to eat, shop, attend shows and concerts, or travel. That would make me angry!

Boredom

Mom's main problem now is her boredom. Few people visit her; seniors seem to be forgotten. My grandparents outlived all their friends. Some of Mom's closest friends are still alive but do not drive; Mom is unable to call them. With her poor eyesight she cannot read, never wanted audio tapes (because she would not admit she is visually impaired), and cannot see or follow the subject on TV any more. My uncle, who always liked sports, also has stopped watching TV. I do not know how to fix their boredom. He does go outside for a daily walk in nice weather and sometimes works on large puzzles. Mom never did crochet, knit, or do crafts. Bingo, church meetings, singers, and entertainers are the only things that perk Mom's interest. The bingo board has large letters and numbers, and they place her bingo chips in a bowl, so she can play with a little help. She has the nurse push re-dial on the phone to call me daily. That does not fill the days, so they both sit in their lobbies and watch people come and go.

When she had a boil recently, they put her to bed for one or two hours during the day to relieve pressure points. She hated that! Now they move her to her recliner in her room for a few hours daily.

Loss and Death

While still at the assisted living, Mom's best friend there, who was in her 90s, broke her hip and moved to another facility, where she died a few months later. Mom missed her immensely. Several of my uncle's male buddies have moved to other facilities with more care. There are only a few men at his assisted living. Many of their long time friends have died. Remember, your parents are facing loss and death often with their aging friends.

15

Emotional Issues for You

Things Will Get Worse.

You must accept that your parents will not get better; in fact, things will get worse.

Your goals must be to:

- Give them the best quality of life.
- Improve your relationship with them.
- Do not ruin your health or marriage.

Keep your sense of humor! Realize this is a temporary situation and will not last forever. It might just seem like forever! Look for humor wherever possible!

One old man said to his buddy, "Do you ever worry about the hereafter?" His friend replied, "Yes, every day I walk into a room and say what am I here after?"

Only Child

The bad news: You do all the work.

The good news: You do not have to share!

As an only child you might feel all the work is dumped on you. You are responsible for your parents; this is true. There are advantages. You make all the decisions and do not have to consult or argue with others about their wants or wishes. You do not expect anyone else to do something and then be disappointed when they do not. You get to keep anything you want from the parents' belongings.

I never minded being an only child. I traveled more places with my parents and was probably closer to my parents. Three of my high school friends were the "only child," and we became close. Today I consider them my adopted "sisters" and a major part of my support system.

One dear friend stayed for all three days of the auction in the 98 degree heat. She and her husband ran errands to save me time. They truly are part of my family and support system! Another dear friend has been my life line throughout my life and is an excellent sounding board. She has listened and offered excellent advice. With my math background I focus on specific details and implementation. She has enabled me to focus on the bigger picture instead of the immediate issue. I probably would have blown my top without her!

Stress

Stress impacts your immune system. Be aware of the stress on your own health in moving the parents, cleaning out, and selling their home. These are significant tasks and may happen in a different order and require months and even years to complete.

There can be stress on you if there is a minor or major change such as a caregiver quits, your parents have an illness or hospital stay, or one dies. One friend shared that she had pain in her neck for several years. Then about six months after her father died, the pain was gone. Another friend suggested it was probably stress over caring for her father and other family responsibilities. (*See* **Take Care of Yourself**.)

Guilt/Shame

Guilt saps your energy and does not accomplish anything. Do not feel guilty! Do not throw guilt to others; do not accept guilt. Do not allow guilt to control your choices. Guilt is a wasted emotion. Brian Tracy says our parents have used guilt for years to control and manipulate us into doing what they want; many are still trying to use it because it worked! Do not allow it anymore.

Did you want to keep your mother at home with your sister and lose your sister's health or sanity? Would your husband leave if your parents moved in? These are difficult questions.

Many children feel guilty about past choices or about moving their parents out of their home or the family home into an assisted living or a skilled care facility. Sometimes siblings have cared for the parents for years and need their lives back, but the children still feel guilty.

Mom chose to stay in her hometown; I chose to stay where my son lives and where I have lived for over thirty years. That does not make either choice wrong.

If we continue to feel guilt and shame over events and keep re-living the past, we will miss enjoying the present. We cannot change the past. Let it go. All we can do is try to learn from our past mistakes, make better choices from today forward, and take action.

"Don't look back because you might fall over what is in front of you." by Kate Williams, age 7. Joel Osteen said the windshield is large, and the rear view mirror is small in a car because it is more important to look forward than back.

You have done the right thing. You are not a bad person for putting your parents in a facility. You are making the best choices you can with the current information. If conditions or circumstances change, you can make another choice for your parents and you. Make choices that give you peace of mind, keep you healthy, and keep your parents safe.

Anger/Rage/Frustrations

Do not allow them to "push your hot buttons."

Why do I have to handle all the messes my mother left? She did not want to do the work. She had so much stuff that it literally took two years to move from one house to the larger house she bought when she was 69. And then she proceeded to fill up the new house. She did not organize, clean out her house, or reduce her belongings. She did not want to take her time to do this or might not have had the energy or motivation. But somebody had to do it!

She would not allow me to draft her bills even though she could not see to write the checks. It was a concern that someone in the office at the assisted living was filling out Mom's checks, and Mom would sign them. She would not give me her checkbook at that time. Hurrah for my online bank access that enabled me to monitor the checks that were written!

Choose your words wisely. Your words have power. Say only what you want to happen. Even with dementia if there is a strong emotion associated with an event, your parents will remember it. If you say something mean or angry that hurts their feelings, they will remember it when they cannot tell you what they had for their last meal. Beware of your tongue and choice of words! They can be as deadly as a sword. Your words determine your future, so use them wisely.

Even now Mom remembers any event tied to money. She remembers what she wins at bingo. Since she thinks her parents died a few months ago, she wants her inheritance!

Anger is a poison that you take, and expect the other person to die.

Anger is a choice. We choose how we react to situations. I did not realize this for a long time: We choose to get angry. Ask yourself, "Is this worth giving up my peace and serenity?" For every minute you are angry or upset, you give up a minute of happiness and peace that you can never get back. I am working to choose happiness and serenity more than I choose anger, but it takes constant work on my part.

Realize you will have disagreements with your parents. Try to resolve issues, so you both win.

I had these thoughts and you might, too:

Why me? There is no one else to do it!

Why do I have to clean out her house? She did not have the energy.

Why am I doing all the work, and she is doing nothing? She is ill with dementia.

Why do I have to handle her business? She cannot do it herself.

Why does she repeat everything five times? Why does she wipe her mouth twenty times? These are signs of dementia.

Why do I have to sell her house? She would not leave it willingly.

Why will she not allow me to draft her bills? She does not do business that way.

Why will she not allow me to go outside after dark at her house? She thinks it is dangerous, and somebody might kidnap me!

Why can I not run errands by myself? She wanted to get out, needed to ensure her business was handled correctly, and had to keep me safe. (Everything takes so much longer when they go with you!)

You can have these thoughts and probably will but do not dwell on them. Your parents did the best they could; now you have to do the best you can with the cards you are dealt. Wishing or complaining will not make the work go away. Think of it as serving God as you work through each item. It will convert your self-pity and anger into realizing you are helping others. My parents never complained when they were raising me about the messes I made or how expensive it was to send me to college. I should not complain now.

Colossians 3:23-24 *Whatever your task, work heartily, as serving the Lord and not men, knowing that from the Lord you will receive the inheritance as your reward; you are serving the Lord Christ.*

She criticized anything I did, so why would I want to do anything for her? For several years Mom seemed to fight me on everything. We just do things differently. That does not make her way or my way wrong. It does make it difficult in trying to please her. You do not feel as if you are getting closure on any issues, and many times you are not. This can be frustrating and discouraging. It takes so much extra time and work. Here is a simple example: I wanted to take the trash out to the street after dark. Mom would not allow me to go outside after dark because it was dangerous. She wanted me to keep the trash inside the house or in my car. She physically blocked me from going out the door. What should have been a simple task was turned into a confrontation!

She needed to watch me all the time; I was not allowed to go out alone. That confirmed we could not co-exist for more extended periods of time together. I moved her back into her house whenever I visited, but her constant fears meant she needed to live in an assisted living the majority of the time.

She did not want me to move any items in her house because it would make a mess, and she certainly did not want to go through any boxes. It was too much work. This meant I could not sort anything while she was in the house.

Once my mother moved into an assisted living, I realized that I could not work outside the home. I needed to clean out her house across 1,000 miles on numerous trips. It took four and a half years to prepare for the three-day auction.

Of course, when I stopped working, Mom wanted me to move into her house and live with her. I knew that was impossible after the battle over the trash. Mom tried to impose her fears on me, and I would not permit it.

Counseling

When you feel overwhelmed, you do not know where to start. In the business world I was a successful manager, who handled large projects. Why was I losing my hair dealing with my aging mother? I was so stressed realizing the amount of work to be done that my hair literally started falling out, and my neck was swollen and sore. I think it was the stress. At this point I knew I needed an outside viewpoint. My company benefits gave eight free counseling sessions per year, so I met with a counselor for help and guidance. I asked her to address the emotional turmoil of dealing with **all my mother's stuff**. The counselor helped me immensely to assess the current situation, to address and prioritize the issues, and to focus on the important things. It just took a few sessions to reset my thoughts and gain a better perspective. It helped to realize others have felt the same way, and there are workable solutions.

These were the counselor's valuable suggestions:

- I am an only child, so I make all the decisions.

- My mother has financial resources, so there is no urgency or deadline in selling the house.

- I can go through things and clean out the house at my own pace. One person who lived six hundred miles away took four years to clean out his parents' house; there does not have to be a deadline.

- Those who do not do, complain. I could never seem to please my mother; she just complained no matter what I did. Either she wanted me to improve and always be better, or it was that I did not do things her way. Sometimes people who do not do, complain in order to put a person down and make themselves feel or look better.

- I did not need to please my mother. She would not be at the house; I would be making the decisions and doing the work.

- I needed to keep Mom happy in a safe environment and have her last days as pleasant as possible. This does not mean I would move to her town. I had not lived in the same town with Mom since high school, but she tried to tie her happiness to my visits.

At work I was accustomed to projects having target completion dates. I had to realize with parent/child relationships there is no closure on this project until both parents die, the estate is handled, and the house is sold. You have no idea if that will last one month or sixteen years. You are in it for the long haul, so pace yourself.

Since Mom was financially sound, there was no rush or deadline for selling her house. I am an only child, so I make all the decisions. This removed a tremendous "unknown" amount of stress. I just needed to treat this like a project at work: plan, implement, and make modifications as needed. I did not add the pressure of a completion date.

Cleaning out her house and my Grandmother's house with my cousins took much **time, sweat, and perseverance.** There were some fun discoveries, but overall it was a great deal of work. My primary reason in completing these major projects was to honor my parents and my Grandmother.

Note: If you are working in basements or moldy, dusty environments, wear a face mask. In working in Grandma's basement I wore a face mask, my cousin did not, and she got a sinus infection.

Mom was not going to change.

If I tried to change her or argue with her, I got frustrated. If we continued down this path, I would go crazy! When I complained to my uncle about Mom's actions, my uncle astutely told me, "Your mother is not going to change." He was right! It took me quite awhile to internalize that she was not going to change, and I just had to deal with those facts. Getting angry was not going to help. I had to quit trying to change her. Finally I realized I had to adapt and change my actions, reactions, choices, and my mindset. People only change if they see some advantage to change, or they are willing to change for someone they love. That was a hard lesson to learn!

At some point, I stopped asking for her permission or approval and just started doing what I thought was the right thing. This was the beginning of my becoming the parent and her becoming the child. I think I had that "aha" moment after I started doing so. It removed much of my stress and emotional turmoil when I took charge just as I was successful doing at my job. When I am doing all the work, it is okay for me to make the decisions as long as I keep her best interests at heart.

Also, Mom is set in her ways and seemed to fight me every step of the way. It is difficult dealing with the status quo, "I've always done it this way." An example is direct deposit. She wanted to see her monthly check before she deposited it in the bank. When she stopped driving, it was difficult to get it deposited in a timely way. She never considered that with direct deposit there is less chance for it being lost, plus it gets in the bank several days sooner. My uncle at almost 89 just agreed to direct deposit for his monthly check recently!

Control

Parents do not like to give up control.

Mom was accustomed to being in control of her house, her belongings, and her money. I was accustomed to being in control of my house, my belongings, and my money along with managing my projects at work. So when she moved out of the house into the assisted living, I started treating her house and belongings as I would mine. Essentially, without fully accepting it, she was giving up control over these things. To our parents, giving up control is just another sign of their decline and lack of freedom.

Forgiveness

Being angry or holding grudges against your parents only hurts you. They might be angry with you for things you have said or done, too, so it is important that you do two things:

- **Ask your parents to forgive you** for anything that hurt them.
- Tell them, **"I forgive you."**

They might not understand what you mean, but it will help you let go of your anger. You do not need to go into specifics; it is probably better if you do not. Your parents did not have an instruction manual on raising children. They did the best they could. You were not always an easy child or teenager! Now they are or will be the "children," and you are or will be the "parent."

Confrontation

Keep this primary goal in mind: safety and well-being of your parents and their finances.

I do not like confrontations; many people do not like to confront or challenge other people about decisions. I like it when everyone is working together toward a common goal for the betterment of all, but I had to confront Mom on two occasions. It was obvious I needed to take over paying her bills. She did not want to give up control of her finances, but lack of bill payment would cause negative consequences. I told her I was paying her bills. She got mad and threw a temper tantrum, but I got the result that needed to happen. I didn't want the work of paying her bills, but it was the right thing to do.

The other time I confronted Mom concerned the auction of her belongings. I came home to have the auction and told her. She replied, "I don't want you to sell my belongings." I told her, "You don't have a choice. I have not rushed into this. You are unable to live in your house and can no longer enjoy them. I have waited four and a half years." She got mad and didn't speak to me initially! She needed my help, attention, and love, so her exterior anger did not last long. Unfortunately, she allowed her mind (her mental state) to make her body physically ill about the auction, so she ended up in the hospital. (*See* **Risks and Choices**.)

One important issue that might require you to confront your

parents involves ending their driving. Their continuing to drive could be dangerous to themselves and others; there is risk of a lawsuit if they cause a serious accident. (*See* **End of Driving**.)

Give a specific topic much thought, consider the consequences of both sides of the issue, and discuss it with a good friend. Sometimes it helps me to take a piece of paper and make two columns for Pros and Cons. Then fill in the items for each column. It is very difficult to confront your parents. They are your parents! They are the authority figures. You respect them. Now it is time for you to become the parent, and you will know the right thing to do. (*See* **Role Reversal**.)

Change of Viewpoint

Sometimes it is helpful to pretend your parents and you are characters in a movie you are watching. Many times I got so emotionally involved that I lost perspective. When you replay the event in your mind as viewed from above, it makes you think about your choice and realize you need to modify it next time.

My Personal Goals for This Transition Period

- Do what I know to be right.
- Choose faith in God and show love; faith and love are the opposite of fear.
- Choose calm and peacefulness.
- Do not allow Mom to control me.
- Do not allow Mom to create fear in me.
- Do not get angry or allow her to sap my energy.
- Do not criticize or correct Mom; her feelings and choices are not wrong.
- Accept who Mom is; she will not change.
- Give true compliments to Mom; validate her.

16

Take Care of Yourself

If you do not take care of yourself, you will not be able to help others.

You must take care of yourself mentally, physically, emotionally, and spiritually. If you do not, the situation will sap your energy, your health, and your life.

Reward yourself for major accomplishments. Buy a dress or a golf club; take a trip. There is much work to be done, so pace yourself for what can be a long journey.

For several years I had not traveled outside the United States since Mom was in the assisted living. My son told me to go on a trip with my girlfriend. I agonized over telling Mom because she gets so worried when I fly and travel on vacation. I did not tell her but told the caregivers that I would be gone for ten days. I prayed she would not die while I was on vacation! When I returned home, Mom was mad that I did not call for several days. She never realized that I was on vacation, out of the country, or gone for ten days! I certainly did not tell her! That trip brightened my outlook, provided wonderful memories, and revitalized me. Vacations are important. They lift off the responsibilities at least for a few days and recharge your batteries.

Find stress relievers. It is important to have stress relievers in a variety of forms to save your sanity. It is critical to your well-being. Take a timeout for yourself; you deserve a break.

Have a life line, someone whom you can call anytime day or night. It is helpful if that person has dealt with an aging parent. It is better to vent to your friend than your sibling or spouse. You need to get your frustrations out verbally (talking or yelling) or physically (walking or exercising), so they do not affect your mental or physical health. I have one dear high school friend who has helped me through many difficult periods of life. Her valuable talent is in listening and being a sounding board. She knew Mom and understands her ways that can frustrate me. I helped her through some difficult times with her aging relatives. We can always tell each other everything and vent, as needed, to keep from blowing our top. She re-focuses me on the goal and the big picture. Many times she will have excellent ideas when I am too close to the problem to see a solution. During some periods we talked multiple times per day. She has saved my sanity and maybe my life.

It would be helpful to have multiple people who have gone through this and could offer you support and insight. Knowing your friends have experienced the same feelings and course of events is comforting. Each has used a different approach, and it helps to realize there are multiple choices. You do not want to wear down your primary life line.

Scream! At times I literally went into the yard and actually screamed as loud as I could. It was such an amazing stress reliever! Before you get to the end of your rope, try it. Or you can scream into a pillow if neighboring houses are near.

Any form of exercise is a stress reliever and good for the body and mind. Exercise creates positive endorphins and serotonin while relieving stress and removing toxins.

Walking is very therapeutic. I found it helpful to pray as I walked, to just enjoy nature, and to be quiet while away from my responsibilities and parent.

Yoga is wonderful for calming the mind as well as exercising and cleansing all parts of the body while building muscle. I used a local exercise facility while I was in my hometown for several months.

Hitting a tennis ball or racquet ball is a wonderful stress release. Even though I did not have a partner while I was in my hometown, I would use the hit wall for tennis practice.

Eat healthy foods. Avoid using food, especially salty, sweet, and fatty items, and alcohol as stress relievers. Beware of how you "feed" your emotions. These will cause other problems later for you. You and your parents need to make healthy food choices.

Have fun! Attend a band concert, go out to eat, or spend time with a friend.

Avoid injuring yourself while helping your parents. Mom gradually moved to using a walker and then had trouble getting up and getting started. When I was there, I would take her to doctors' appointments, friends' homes, the hair salon, and restaurants often, but this required I assist her into and out of the car and getting up from the chair. She weighs about 160 pounds. I had injured my knee playing sports, but on one trip after helping her get up multiple times and hearing my knee crunch, I required surgery to remove torn cartilage.

You need boundaries. Especially when your parents live with you, you need to set boundaries about what and when you will do things for them, what you expect them to do for themselves, and how often they accompany you on outings. You need time with your spouse and your friends, so do not allow them to totally consume you.

These boundaries are even necessary if they live in a facility in your town. They might expect you to visit every day at a set time, but you probably should vary the time for your visits.

17

Friends' Situations

A friend's mother had a serious staph infection at age 52 when her daughter was 12. The daughter had to step up and do many household chores since her mother was not very mobile with her leg brace and crutches. At age 14 her father had a stroke, so in many ways, the daughter became an adult at that time. The mother was widowed early, and my friend, an only child, was responsible for helping her mother. For some years the daughter lived in a house near her mother's home. As the mother got older, she moved to different parts of the country in assisted living facilities as the daughter and husband moved with his work. She realized the benefits of being near her daughter and grandchildren and having her daughter visit daily. When she moved to California, she exchanged her dresses for slacks to stay up to date! The mother lived to be 98, and the daughter finished well by providing excellent, loving care for her mother although it was extremely difficult and time consuming for such an extended period of time.

One friend visited her parents for a week and stayed a month when her father became ill and died. Her rental car bill was ridiculous, but she did not have a choice.

One friend sacrificed her friendships and life to care for her aging mother for many years. She felt this was the right choice for her mother and her. She moved into her mother's home and gave up her job the last year of her mother's life, but it saved the major expense of a facility. (We never know how long our parents will live.) After her mother's death it took her almost a year to clean out the mother's house and prepare for an estate sale. During her years of service she fed her emotions with sweet treats, stopped exercising, and gained a significant amount of weight. Now she is dealing with the emotional trauma of not having a social life and the health impacts of her weight. Her mother has been dead for two years, and the house has just sold, so she will finally get closure on the estate.

One friend's mother had Alzheimer's disease and was initially placed in a skilled care facility near one daughter. Amazingly, she retained her piano playing skills. She was a very capable, strong willed woman; falls and broken bones did not deter her. She remained quite mobile. Through the years she was moved to different facilities to be close to one daughter in Missouri, another daughter in Georgia, and then a third daughter in Illinois. She had been a home economics teacher and practiced excellent nutrition throughout her life. She lived to be 96.

One friend's sister was living with her mother for many years but could not continue caring for her. The last several years they hired help to stay in the house during the day with their mother. Then the sister just could not do it anymore. My friend was so upset and felt so guilty about putting her mother in a facility at 90, but they had to think about the sister's well-being. They delayed it as long as possible, but the sister needed to get her life back. She had put it on hold for many years just as my other friend did for her mother. Their mother did not make it easy by refusing to get out of the car and go in the facility. The facility knows what to do to help their mother. She might not like it now, but I hope she will adjust. (*See* **Friends' Shared Feelings**.)

One friend had 24-hour care for her mother in her parents' home for several years. Her father was still living but was unable to perform the amount of care required. This was very expensive and also took much time for planning, hiring, managing, and paying help in the home. For these reasons when they realized their father required assistance, she and her sisters decided to move him into a nice assisted living. He was not eating well and could not remember how things worked in the house. His safety was their main concern. They had investigated places and talked with their father for a year before the change occurred. Their father never accepted nor adjusted to his new environment even though it was an excellent facility. He was unwilling to socialize there. It did not matter that his daughters visited and called often. Our parents are unhappy leaving their homes, but we know they cannot return. No matter what choice you make, it is difficult emotionally on them and you. Most will adjust; some never do.

One couple moved to Florida for the warm weather and cheaper housing costs. The couple was very close and loving. When the husband died, I thought the wife might give up and die a few months later. Thankfully, she did not and a year later decided to move to the town where her three sons lived. She has enjoyed many wonderful years with her children and grandchildren. She survived open heart surgery several years ago. At 87 she goes to Curves several times per week and is already working on the Christmas ornaments she makes for her grandchildren every year. She is a positive, loving inspiration to us all.

One friend's brother had his mother living with him. He lifted her so many times that he seriously injured his shoulder and required surgery. His wife developed migraine headaches from the trauma of having the mother living with them. They recently have gotten in-home care to assist them.

One couple sold their house and downsized to a condominium in their mid-70s. She continued to live there after he died. She has broken her hip twice but is a very determined person. She worked through physical therapy and now walks with a cane. She moved into assisted living for short periods during her recoveries. Several months ago, at about 92, she left her condo for a nice assisted living small apartment with three meals per day. She played bridge weekly until recently.

Another family friend at about 85 sold her house, downsized her belongings, and moved into a new independent senior apartment complex that serves two meals a day. Additional services are available, as needed, for nursing care, showering, etc. She has successfully lived there for about six years.

One friend's mother is 95 and almost blind due to macular degeneration. She sold her home after her husband died, and so far is able to live in a senior independent living center with her meals provided. Her son lives nearby and is able to check on her regularly.

One family friend stayed in her house with her son until she was about 92. She still drove and played bridge weekly. Then she moved to a skilled care facility for about two years until she died last year.

At about 88, another family friend bought the small ranch style house she lived in as a newlywed and downsized her belongings. At 90 she is still driving and active playing the piano to perform for her music club.

One church widow friend in her 70s moved into an apartment and is an active volunteer at the hospital gift shop and delivers Meals on Wheels. Her healthy habit is to eat blueberries daily.

A couple of years ago one church friend, who was about 85 and a widower, sold his home and used the money to buy into a nice assisted living facility. He plays bridge once a week, participates in other activities there, and still attends church. He recently went on a seniors' trip to New England with his church buddies. This World War II pilot and POW still drives locally and seems happy with his choice.

One church woman recently admitted she is 86. She ushers every Sunday, helps prepare the Wednesday church suppers, and volunteers at the city senior center one day a week. She owns a cabin in the mountains and visits it often. She clearly stated, "It will kill me to stop driving and lose my independence."

After her elderly mother and husband died, my aunt bought a

small ranch style house where she lived until she was 92. She remained active cutting her grass and still driving. She was in a skilled care facility for about three months before she died.

One aunt died at 87 in her own home. She had breast cancer in her fifties but was a long-term survivor.

At about 85 my uncle was living alone in his house but was cooking less as indicated by his losing weight and having less food in his refrigerator. To supplement his nutrition he started getting Meals on Wheels once daily Monday through Friday. He limited his driving to short distances to meet friends for breakfast, attend church, and get groceries. He was once hospitalized for some heart issues then returned home. About a year later he had a minor heart attack one evening and spent the night on the kitchen floor. When his daughter called in the morning and did not get an answer, she alerted her brother to check on him. At that point the doctor and his children knew he needed to move to an assisted living. His facility is very pleasant, and he says the food is really good. I know it smells good when I visit! For several months he wanted to get his car and go home. His children sold his car at Mom's auction, and he was not happy about it. He finally accepted he needs to stay and now seems content. He is almost 89 with some short-term memory issues but overall is in good health. There are not many men in his facility. His good buddy, who needed more care, recently moved to Mom's facility. The faces change over time as people die, move to a skilled care facility, or recover from a health issue and move back home. Previously he was a sports enthusiast, but lately he does not watch TV. He reads the newspaper daily and always checks the obituaries "to make sure my name isn't listed!" He still has his good sense of humor! He was always active and slim, and he still takes walks with his walker around the parking lot. Since his walker goes on pavement, I replaced his worn out plastic skis. He has two children who work in the same town, so they check on him regularly. Another daughter lives in a neighboring state and comes about every eight weeks to take him to doctors' appointments, get his hair cut, check on his clothes, and take him to the podiatrist. The adult children are currently making repairs to his home but have not put it on the market.

When I was in Missouri recently, a 102-year-old woman walked with a cane into the restaurant and joined us for lunch. She is quite sharp and belongs to my friend's church.

One friend's mother had a stroke soon after her father retired. The father became very angry because he wanted to travel and enjoy his retirement but could not with his wife disabled in a wheelchair. He had taken in his in-laws during their senior years and expected one of his children to do the same. The children felt their mother needed too much care. This couple was inseparable, so they moved to a facility together. She was very social and adapted well to her new environment, but he never did. He had worked very hard his whole life, saved his money, and looked forward to retirement. His dream for retirement never materialized, and he remained angry. After his wife died, he just willed himself to die.

A woman who lives at Mom's facility had a stroke or some disabling event and is unable to converse or feed herself. Her husband of 53 years comes almost daily to eat supper with his wife. He shared their story. His wife initially went to an assisted living facility for 39 days, but it did not provide enough care. He moved her to a skilled care facility. There was an attempted rape of her roommate by a male living in the facility, so he quickly moved her to another facility. One day he visited her during lunch time; his wife only had on a blouse, and the aides had gone to the lunchroom without her. He moved her to her current facility and is very pleased with his wife's care. His words of advice were sometimes it takes awhile to find the right place. That was a comfort to me that he plans to leave his wife at Mom's facility.

One friend in her mid-60s, who had both knees replaced, downsized her belongings, sold her house, and moved into a large four-bedroom condominium. Now she does not have any yard work and can easily travel many months per year to visit her children and vacation. She just locks the door and leaves.

18

Friends' Shared Feelings

My GA Friend moved her mother, who lived in her family home with the other daughter, into a skilled care facility. This prompted a sharing of e-mail messages from our dear college friends regarding dealing with aging parents.

GA Friend

"We are busy getting things figured out here. I will go…and my sister and I will put my mom into a skilled nursing home. A room became available this week. My mom has taken a turn and is much less aware of "things" and is a challenge daily, so it is time. My poor sister has been shouldering all of this, and she needs her life back. It is time, but I'm not saying that will make it any easier.

"Just to make all this even more exciting, my husband's previous boss called and wants him to work in NYC for awhile. He wanted us to move there. My husband does not want that but said he would go help out. He leaves Mon. They rented him a corp. apt. in SoHo, and he will be off on his adventure. They were talking months; now it is sounding more like weeks. I do not know. It is what it is. It would be fun to have a weekend up there with him. The girls were very excited.

"Well, it is a sad, crazy, busy time here."

"Well, we made the big move today; she did not kick and scream, but it was still very difficult. We arrived at the place, and once she saw it, she said she was not getting out of the car. Suddenly, she was not at all confused. We were able to get her inside and to her room. We then distracted her with an activity, and my sister and I unpacked her clothes and set up her room. She was not even aware we brought all her stuff.

"After the activity we stayed with her for dinner; it went okay. The trouble started when we said she had to walk down this long hall back to 'her room.' She said, 'Do not call it that.' She was having NO part in having a room there. She did not want to walk that far, so when she passed an empty wheel chair, she sat down in it.

"It was clearly going to be a Mexican stand-off. I went out and talked to the night nurse, a very nice guy. I told him she was refusing to do anything and did not want to see where her stuff was. He said I am going to tell you something you do not want to hear. I said you are going to tell us to leave. He smiled and said, 'Go, she will be fine.' I motioned to my sister, we said good-bye, we will see you tomorrow with a stiff upper lip, and we were out the door. We called after 11, were told she watched TV (she would not do that when we were there), and was asleep.

"We really have this feeling tomorrow will be worse. My sister has come down with a cold tonight. I hope she does not feel too bad tomorrow. We all need to sleep, that I know for sure.

"We will take more photos, etc., tomorrow."

"We came home and started throwing away stuff from her room.... There is lots of junk, but a few minor treasures like my dad's school pin. We were actually looking for a MISSING RING; I think that is long gone. We have so much trash and items for goodwill. That felt good, but we are still in the mess stage before it actually looks better. I just wanted to help my sister as much as I can before I leave.

"My husband is in NYC working. I'm glad he had some company; he had a hard week.

"Okay, going to sleep. Thanks so much for all the good thoughts, moral support, and good wishes.

"Love,

"GA Friend"

∽ఎ ౬∾

"I am on my way home on the plane now. Hopefully I will successfully save and be able to send this later. Thank you all for your calls and e-mail messages. They are/were much appreciated. I am sorry I could not respond to everyone, but way too stressed, tired, and busy most of the time.

"I am still processing all that went on. My sister, my brother, and I were a team. Naturally my sister had to be the one to do the interviews and advance visits. She and I had gone to see this particular place over a year ago. She did visit several more to make sure.

"The staff seems pretty responsive. Naturally we care more than they do, so we are trying not to sweat the small stuff.

"Each day she has demanded to go home. That is hard. Some days were worse than others."

✨

"I think everything hit me when I was on my way home. Once here I feel even more guilty and helpless. When I was there, we were doing so much in the house, I guess we were distracted. If my ticket had not been so expensive already, and if my husband were not coming home Friday, I probably would have stayed longer.

"We have taken a ton of junk out of the house. We cleaned closets and got bags and bags for donation. We have floor guys lined up for tomorrow to take off two layers of tile in the hall. We are hoping the hardwoods underneath will be able to be salvaged. My mom's bedroom carpet is history; next is refinishing. The floor guys will take out carpet from another bedroom/office and refinish my sister's exposed hardwood to match. What a huge project to empty all those closets and move furniture.

"I spent a lot of time rearranging the kitchen and bringing up my sister's stuff that has been in boxes for 10 years. We did the rest of the house every day when we were at home. Kitchen was worked on midnight to about 2 AM a few nights in a row. Sleeping was not on the schedule. Needless to say we got a lot of major stuff either started or done, but more remains. We have electrical and major painting. Not even thinking about the hardwood floors in the living room and dining room under old carpeting. Doing one or two things just leads to the next. It is a journey. I needed to paint, but there was no time.

"My mom wants out. It tears me apart. I had to call her lifelong best friend and tell her. That is when I really lost it. She saw us all with my mom at the beauty shop the day we made the move. We could not tell her anything in front of my mom. When I called her, she said she knew. She did not sleep the night she saw us; she had figured it out. She lives in a seniors' high-rise, is several years older than my mom, but is sharp.

"CA Friend, NC Friend, and MOA Friend, I'm not sure how you

did this. I know MOB Friend has had these issues to deal with, too, and MOC Friend will soon. The idea and the place is not so bad, it is how the person does with things, how social they are, and their general health and mental condition.

"I think a lot of tears are yet to be. It is sad for her for sure.

"My husband will be back Fri. evening. He is in DC working for 2 days. He could not have been more supportive. He wants me to go back to NYC with him sometime next week. I cannot even think right now.

"Dogs and I will start walking again tomorrow, rain or shine. Start walking and stop eating is the plan. They were so excited when I got home, but I could tell they were looking for my husband, too. I think, I know, he is their first choice.

"Okay, good night all. I am sure my mom and I will have our good and bad days. That's true for my sister and brother, too. Our daughters have promised to shoot us when we get to this stage. This aging thing sucks!

"Love you all, **we need to fill up on life while we still can.**"

"Well, I'm still home playing catch up and trying to come to terms with my mom's situation. She does not have a phone (she had given up talking on the phone anyway), but my sister let her talk to me on her cell after I left. She gave me a boat load of unhappy, mad, frustrated....

"I hope all are well and finding something fun to do, too! It is time we enjoy ourselves. I had an e-mail from our high school class; it was death notices of 3 classmates. Two were heart, and one was cancer. *Fill up on life...words to live by! No one has promised us tomorrow. I just had a friend die after a 5 year struggle with cancer at age 60.*"

"My mom was on a walker and is still using that in her room but uses a wheel chair to get to any activity, etc. She is not too steady on her feet."

"The phone and my mom — well, she has not been talking on the phone for about 6 months. It is harder and harder to talk to her on the phone. She gave up calling even her sister about a year ago even with her phone number on a white erase board posted in the kitchen. She wants no part of it. I have my sister there to visit and see her, so no phone in theory is frustrating for out of town family but in reality is probably okay. The 2 minutes I was on the phone with her she dragged me right down, and I felt awful instantly. I am pretty good at doing that all by myself.

"She already fell but was not hurt. I know that happens, look at MOA Friend's mom, I think she fell in each place."

MOA Friend

"CA Friend, you asked how I'm doing (since my mother's death). I am saddened almost every morning by realizing again that she is gone. I think back and picture her as she was when I was younger. I remember her strength and her capability. It makes me feel sad, and it also makes me feel very 'non-grounded.' Somehow I don't feel as much a part of the whole big world anymore. I think I feel I'm on that down-hill side of things, but I still intend to enjoy what I have left.

"Facing the fact that we are the next 'disappearing generation' is a bit thought provoking. I think I feel scared for my children more than anything. I guess I don't want them to be here by themselves in case they need me to buffer for them. But I know they will do fine as we all did.

"We can all think about this and how it makes us feel, and then we look around us and 'go on.' We cannot change the natural process of life/death, and although we've always known that, it's becoming more and more obvious.

"Looking back, I feel very lucky to have lived in the era we did live in. What great childhoods we had. I hope that our kids feel the same, but I know ours were best!

"I hope that MOB Friend, GA Friend, NC Friend, and MOC Friend still have some quality time with your parent. All I can say is to try to value being able to look at them, touch them, and talk with them. Know that you must make decisions that they are not comfortable with in the interest of keeping them safe. Placing them where other people are always close is a safety issue and is the best that we can do.

"Looking back, I wish that I had asked more about my parents' early life – the 'history of them', some questions about recipes, and many questions about WW II for my dad."

MOB Friend

"All of your notes have been so encouraging, and we learn from each other. It makes me appreciate each of your friendships even more.

"GA Friend, your current situation took me back to dealing with my elderly uncle for several years. Near the end when he had just had a test that determined he could no longer swallow correctly due to mini-strokes, he looked me right in the eye one morning and said, 'TAKE ME HOME!' I was so saddened (plus felt guilty) because I knew it wasn't possible at that point, and he only lived a few more days. The interesting thing was we had taken him back to his house just a few weeks before when he had a doctor's appointment. He didn't recognize anything on that visit, nor did he remember he had even been there 30 minutes afterward! I think he was really stressed by that point in time. We had to concentrate on the good times and even humorous ones, such as one night when he wrote a letter of resignation to the director of the nursing home! He was adamant about delivering it that night, and we were so lucky to have an understanding night nurse who came to our rescue.

"I also recall my mother telling my dad and us she just wanted to go home one more time when she was in the hospital for the last time. It broke our heart (and I'm tearing up right now writing this) not to be able to fulfill that wish.

"And then last year in the span of a month and a half, we had our youngest son's wedding, our oldest son had his third surgery, and then we had to help put my stepmother into a nursing home and my dad into assisted living. Talk about an emotional roller coaster! It is so hard to make the difficult decisions in life.

"GA Friend, I do hope you feel up to going to NYC next week for a little R & R with your husband. It may be good to have a change of scenery. It does sound as if you three accomplished so much. My dad's situation made it easier since they moved from our family home to Jonesboro (and downsized), then moved to independent living (downsizing again), and then he went to assisted living. There aren't many things left. Now I'm thinking like CA Friend. I know how much stuff we have in our own house and have started to purge.

"I need to end here and decide if I'm going to a basketball game tonight with my husband and our neighbor. Dinner needs to come first, too. Thanks for all of your caring thoughts and words."

꧁ ꧂

MOC Friend

"Some of you asked how my mother is doing. Mom, at age 95, is doing really well, but she is definitely slowing down and showing some signs of memory loss. I call her 4 times a day to be sure she takes her medications (for heart and macular degeneration). Most of the time she remembers but has 'off' days, so I can't assume she will remember.

"We probably will need to look at assisted living (in our home or at another facility) sometime in the near future, I think. Meanwhile, we try to take her out to eat and to the store and beauty shop several times a week. We will take her and her 100-year-old girlfriend (who is in GREAT shape) to breakfast on Monday!

"I try to go see Mom at least once a day, and we do everything at random times to keep her out of too much of a mental routine and to minimize boredom. She can still read, which is a real blessing, and she still does exercises every day (mostly sitting down and on her bed since her balance is not great), including riding a daily mile on a stationary bike that she has in her 2-bedroom/2-bathroom independent living apartment. And she tries to eat nutritiously, too. She has lost some weight, so she has been drinking a Boost or Ensure every day. I seriously doubt that I will be in as good condition if I make it to 95!

"We are trying to enjoy every moment we can while we can. She is very careful to have a grateful and thoughtful-about-others attitude regarding her age-related decline. She comments about her awareness of her loss of memory and is sometimes very tired. On the days when she shows signs of memory loss and has occasionally struggled with a bad day, I can see an awareness and fear in her. I see the potential for a tendency toward a rebellion (due to the fear) toward change, even though she told me several years ago that she wants to be put in a nursing home if/when she is 'out of it.'

"It took us more than a year to clean out her house and transition to the independent living apartment. And we were fortunate that she could help us go through everything, and she could afford to wait to sell the house for a while in case she changed her mind. It was the ideal situation, but it was still exhausting for all of us mentally and physically. GA Friend, you and your sister accomplished an unbelievable amount of work while you were there. You must be so exhausted.

"You have all been in my prayers as you have dealt with your situations with your parents. Each of us has to approach this time of life from our unique perspective. You are such dear friends, and you continue to hold a special place in my heart. Thank you all for sharing your hearts and wisdom in this life experience. It is not easy, but we each need to make the difficult decisions based on what is the best for our loved ones, including our spouses and children and siblings, as well as taking into consideration our own health. You have all done admirably in my opinion, and I thank each of you for your example."

19

Moving to Their New Home

It is hard work for you to select what to move and move it.

It is time to downsize their belongings. Do this gradually as they prepare to move.

Do not tell them initially what it costs to live in their new home.

It is scary for your parents to move; they probably have not moved for decades. They might not know anyone at the new place.

This is a difficult transition for your parents. They are angry with you for taking away their independence. One parent refused to get out of the car! One parent had to be tricked to going in. They might complain for days or weeks.

It is helpful if the parents are still sharp enough to make new friends, and their judgment is good enough to understand they needed to move for their own safety and well-being.

Once the parents have moved, they might realize how:

- Much easier life is with someone else doing all the chores like laundry, groceries, meals, and dishes.
- Lonely they were in their house.

- Much they enjoy having company.

- Afraid they were at night that they might fall and not be found quickly.

- Fearful they were to take baths or showers.

In most cases it will be a big relief. But they probably will never admit it to you!

It is not easy physically, mentally, or emotionally moving your parents out of their home to an assisted living or skilled care facility (nursing home). It might have been your home, too. Moving is a big job for anybody. Make all your checklists. After the move it is helpful if a sibling can check on their condition and the food. The quality of the food is almost as important as the care since that is the only thing your parents have to look forward to each day.

I hope your parents do not fight you about this. Some parents do not cooperate or adjust well to changes. It will be hard on you emotionally and physically with all that needs to be done. Some adult children feel guilty, but when you reach this point, you have reviewed the options and made the best decision for their safety and well-being. Be kind to yourself.

If a sibling has been caring for the parents, do not allow it to jeopardize their well-being. Look for signs that it is time to move the parents. Do not feel guilty about it. You must put the well-being of your sibling ahead of your parents because, hopefully, your sibling has a much longer life to live.

Parents can make some good friends at assisted living and enjoy conversations with people their age.

Carefully consider what items your parent will want in their new home, and what will fit in the smaller space. If they do not have room for the family heirlooms, you or your siblings should keep them.

Phone

I recommend you get a phone for their new place with their same phone number, if possible, so friends can call. Mom kept her same number and has a regular phone with large numbers; one friend got her parents a cell phone. I talk to Mom almost daily.

For many years Mom called me three or four times per day; I answered the phone if I was available. Now Mom cannot dial or see the speed dial numbers, so the aides push re-dial to call me. You might not want to hear what they have to say when they first move, but you can tell so much by the sound of their voice. At this point Mom only stays on the phone a few minutes, but I know she is coherent and okay. There are limited things I can ask her, but I can mention bingo on Mondays and Thursdays and church on Sundays. She likes for me to tell her what I have been doing, so she can live vicariously through me. She remembers to ask about her grandson!

Items to Move

Obviously if they are moving to an apartment, they can keep more belongings than if they are moving to one room in a skilled care facility.

Do your parents have recliners or special chairs they like to sit in? Take a few pieces of furniture, so it makes them feel at home. I suggest you move these items:

- Comfortable chair, preferably a recliner for each parent

    At some point you might need to buy them a lift chair that provides an assist in getting up.

- Chair(s) for guests
- End table(s)
- Small dining table (optional) with one or two chairs
- Phone with large numbers
- Lamp(s)

- Wall clock with big numbers and hands
- TV
  Cable is usually not included in the cost but is available for a small fee.
- Bed and appropriate linens if not provided
- Chest or dresser for folded clothes
- Knick knacks or mementoes
- Pictures for the wall to make them feel like home
- Pictures of your parents when they were younger, siblings, and grandchildren as reminders of their family and history
- List of important phone numbers
- Phone book
- Calendar with large numbers
- Paper and pens

Remove the valuables, so they do not "walk away." I have said this multiple times, but too many people have made this mistake, and rings are missing. Keep all gold, valuable jewelry, and furs at home. You do not want to tempt the people working at these facilities, plus it would be upsetting if the expensive items disappeared. Women seem to be okay with a plain gold wedding band. Mom still wants to wear jewelry every day. Since she has a nickel allergy, I get her sterling silver earrings, but several pairs have disappeared. Glass and crystal beads are in style, so I got her several pairs of these. I do not buy pierced earrings with separate backs because they are too hard for the aides to handle. Mom was begging for her diamond ring on my last visit, but it would be gone in hours. She has fake diamond rings that she wears, but I noticed several of her fake diamond rings with sterling mountings are missing now.

Reduce their wardrobe to things that fit and still look nice. Move all their clothes and shoes. I had to get a strong, portable clothes closet because Mom had twice as many clothes as their closet space allowed! I found a nice looking portable, **sturdy** wardrobe at the Container Store where I live and shipped it to her. The first one I bought collapsed!

Label every item of clothing with permanent marker. Pick a unique set of initials or name. I use "C. EDW" for Mom because several people have her last name. The laundry ladies have a tough job. Each visit I go through Mom's closet and return to the front desk items that do not belong to her. Also, periodically they put the "lost" items in the foyer, and I search through those for Mom's missing clothes.

Label your parents' canes, walkers, wheelchairs, leg attachments, wheelchair cushions, and padding with permanent marker. These can easily get mixed up with the others in the facility.

All clothes should be washable. I left a good wool afghan and removed that after the first time they washed it in hot water. Mom's bras just fall apart from the harsh detergents and bleaches, so I started reinforcing them with a soft polyester material, which has lengthened their life.

Warm afghans or throws are needed since your parents are not as active. I got Mom two nice soft, warm afghans and clearly embroidered her label on them. They were missing when I visited in October. I checked Mom's room, the laundry room, and all the storage closets. I did make a fuss over these, so everyone knew they were missing. The laundry lady was upset, so I had to comfort her and tell her she had a tough job. I told her I would buy two more and not to worry about it. By her reaction I did not think she had taken them! Then I purchased two more afghans in a different color (so I will know if the previous ones turn up) and embroidered her label on them. These have stayed in her room.

A humidifier is needed in Mom's room because the dry air in the winter bothers Mom's nose, so I purchased one for her room. The aides keep it filled with water.

Do not let your parents ruin your health, your marriage, or your life.

Your health is the most important thing. My girlfriend had a stroke while she was moving her aging mother to her town. Selling the house, deciding what to move, cleaning out the house, etc., was just too much stress. Remember to keep things in perspective. Realize when you are trying to accomplish too much in too short a time.

Beware of injuring yourself when trying to help parents move from place to place. I no longer offer to help move Mom, and let the aides do the lifting.

Sometimes one facility has assisted living in one section and skilled care in another section. This makes the transition easier on you.

20

Caregiver from a Distance

Pick your battles with the skilled care facility carefully. Do not sweat the small stuff. You do not want to alienate the staff or have them take your complaints out on your parents. I have complained twice in writing about the food. Another issue is they will not order prescriptions via the mail, which would save Mom money. I just found out that her prescription insurance company will not mail drugs to skilled care facilities.

Even if your parents are in a care facility, they still require a significant amount of your time and effort to keep things moving smoothly. There is still a burden or yoke on your shoulders. It is not easy being a caregiver from a distance.

It is expensive for me to fly or drive a 1000 miles three or four times per year. It costs $600–$700 per trip for airfare, rental car, and meals out. For now, I have a place to stay, so that does not include hotel costs. This adds over $2,500 to my annual budget. Sometimes Mom offers to pay for the airfare but not always.

Take funeral clothes with you on visits in case your parents, other family members, or their friends die.

Be aware that going home three to four times per year, taking time to clean out houses, handling her financial affairs, maintaining her house, being available if her house sells, or she gets seriously ill disrupts your focus on a job or career. Mainly for these reasons I have not worked outside the home for five and a half years.

It is always a big relief to get Mom's taxes done each year. This year I did hers and mine in February in case I needed to leave unexpectedly. Even though the heavy weight of the auction has been lifted off my shoulders, I still feel in limbo not knowing when I will get a call, need to go to Missouri on short notice, and possibly stay for an extended time. I still have the responsibility of maintaining her house and am trying to sell it. I am trying to decide whether to get a job.

Daily, monthly, or annually, I:

- Handle all her mail.

- Deposit dividend checks.

- Pay Mom's bills for her skilled care facility, prescriptions, gas, electric, water, yard maintenance, house repairs, insurance, property taxes, Federal and State taxes.

- Balance her checkbook and transfer money as needed.

- Maintain her home.

- Manage her assets and meet with her financial advisor.

- Have discussions with the skilled care facility on Mom's health when they call with any concerns, changes, or medicine changes.

- Communicate with the doctor, as needed, though usually the facility works directly with him.

- Select her annual insurance choices for medical and prescriptions in addition to Medicare and set up payments. This can be time-consuming to fax POA, set up drafts, explain Mom lives in one state, and my mailing address is a different state, etc.

- Collect the information, have her Federal and State taxes

figured by H & R Block in Missouri since they know the state rules, and mail in her tax forms. Completing this from a distance is more difficult, but the local people know Mom and me and are very helpful. I tip the lady who handles Mom's taxes, so she remembers me.

- Send Mom cards for Valentine's, Easter, Mother's Day, Birthday, Anniversary, and Christmas with gifts for several occasions.
- Talk to Mom almost daily.
- Ensure she has a door decoration appropriate for the season, especially for Christmas.

It seems there is something almost daily that I need to handle for Mom, such as her mail, bills, finances, assets, or papers to file. I was already handling these things for my household, so there was no learning curve; it is just extra work.

One year I ordered a special cake, had it delivered to her facility, and invited her dearest friends to attend a gathering for her birthday. Her friends realized that it took me effort and expense to have the celebration, but Mom complained that I was not there. They know it is expensive for me to visit her. Her attitude ruined what could have been a happy event. I will admit that I do not go to Missouri necessarily when *she* wants. I do not like to travel over Christmas and New Year's because of the usual weather concerns and the large volume of travelers. I plan my trips when I can do activities with my college and high school friends, so I can enjoy activities outside the skilled care facility environment. I alternate pleasure with chores because the skilled care facility can be depressing and draining.

Realize that men do not often recognize what needs to be done to care for a mother.

As long as possible, take your parents out to eat, to visit family and friends, to attend musical concerts, to shop, to go for rides, and to attend church.

Every time I visit Mom, I:

- Cut her hair.

- Polish her fingernails.

- Cut her toenails – even though a podiatrist comes regularly to the skilled care facility, they still need trimming and filing.

- Check her clothes for spots, stains, and wear.

- Check her clothes to see if she needs a different size. Mom's clothing size has changed multiple times during her stay in assisted living where it went down and is now going up since she is in a wheelchair. I buy a larger size clothing to allow room for the adult diapers and to make it easier for the aides to quickly pull her slacks down and up while they hold her, and since she is seated all the time, it does not matter if they are a little baggy.

- Check her closet for other people's clothes.

- Check the "lost" items in the lobby for Mom's clothes.

- Check for wounds on her body and especially her feet since she is diabetic. One time she had a wound on her shin that was infected; sometimes their legs get bumped into tables or doorways.

- Check that she has her two afghans.

- Check if the humidifier is working and/or needs cleaning in the winter months.

- Deposit her bingo winnings in her "trust" account for meals out.

- Organize her jewelry, untangle necklaces, and see what she needs as some items might have disappeared.

- Buy her some new clothing items and hose – she still enjoys wearing pretty clothes and jewelry, and though she might not remember if they are new, she knows when she looks nice.

- Check her shoes.

- Check with the facility to learn if she needs any over-the-counter supplements or anything. It is cheaper for me to buy them at Walmart than have them ordered from the pharmacy with other drugs.

- Take her to see her brother. The aides lift her into the car, then I drive her to her brother's assisted living home, and he comes out to see her in the car.

- Take her for a ride around town.

- Bring in her favorite foods, such as ice cream. She loves McDonald's hot fudge sundaes, and at almost 92, I let her enjoy any food she wants.

- Be at her table for at least one meal per day to see the quality of food, how well she can eat by herself, and the quantity of food she eats. She always wants me to eat with her, but the food is not that appealing.

- Host a dinner party for her friends to eat at her skilled care facility in a private room – usually KFC with boneless chicken meals and multiple sides for her and her five friends. The last time I hosted this event, four of them were over 90 and had known each other since high school. I decided not to schedule this during my last visit because she is having trouble eating and chewing and is less able to converse.

- Have financial reviews with appropriate contacts, as needed.

- Check on the house she still owns. I live in it when I visit, so I can ensure everything is in working order.

- Clean the house's yard and gutters of debris.

- Remove the leaves and sticks from the yard.

- Have the debris hauled off.

- Sweep sidewalks and driveways; vacuum the carpet.

- Hold an open house.

- Continue to go through the remaining boxes at Mom's house.

If your parents complain about pain or a fall, check their body and ask questions.

Do things to brighten their days with visits, flowers, gifts, balloons, and treats!

Give flowers to the living. Do not wait and send them to funerals.

While in my hometown I visit my uncle, who lives in an assisted living and is almost 89. He has finally accepted that he needs to stay at the facility. I offer to get him what he needs or wants. One time I got his watch battery replaced. Another time I replaced the plastic pieces on the feet of his walker since it required pliers and a screwdriver. Several times he asked me to bring him beer! Since I am not a beer drinker, I asked what brand he wanted: Pabst Blue Ribbon! Well, I went to the nearby fancy grocery store, which did not carry it. I took him Busch, but I could tell he was disappointed. I looked at another store and found the PBR! I did not ask permission from the facility and brought a 12-pack in a bag and put in his refrigerator. I do not consider him a problem drinker! He has always enjoyed flowers, so this spring I bought a large pot of geraniums and placed them outside the back entrance in his daily view. I thought it might give him something to do in keeping them watered. People have complimented him on his pretty flowers, which brought him some attention, too.

When my older uncle was in a skilled care facility, I would buy him socks and house shoes (washable ones). Label everything you take! These items get lost in the laundry or misplaced. Sometimes I would bring him candy bars since he was not given treats, and he had no way to buy them. He had some missing teeth, so he trained me to not buy any with nuts. When his roommate moved out with his TV, we bought him a TV; that was his only entertainment.

In my hometown I visit many elderly people like Mom's distant cousin, several family friends, and some church friends. These people are in their 90s and seem so glad to see me. I usually attend Mom's church, so the preacher and members will remember who I am. Then I can tell Mom about her friends and family. Also, I visit our family friends who live at Mom's facility. On a recent visit I brought in bouquets of lilacs from Mom's yard. Sometimes I go to the farmers' market and get flowers for their meal tables or buy a flowering potted plant that will last several weeks. These people are lonely and have few visitors, so they appreciate any attention or conversation. Sometimes I play church hymns on the piano at meal times. People appreciate music even if I make some mistakes.

The summer I drove to my hometown and spent almost four months there preparing for the three-day auction of Mom's belongings, I kept enough things in her house for survival living: two folding chairs, card table, lamp, clock, a few pans, a few dishes, glasses, silverware, a microwave, air mattress, sheets, blankets, and towels. I also kept a few tools like gloves, broom, dustpan, vacuum cleaner, rake, hedge trimmer, extension cord, screwdrivers, hammer, caulk gun, caulk, plastic bags, flash light, etc.

While I am in town, I bring Mom food treats, like ice cream and boneless fried chicken. I buy fresh fruits at the farmers' market and bring these for Mom and her table mates. You do need to be aware of food restrictions or allergies for these other people. Fresh fruit tastes so good to them.

I took Mom's favorite foods for supper on my last visit, and she did not handle the situation well. She did not understand why I had spent money when she had food to eat, kept asking what the food was, and where did I get it. It was like a tape that played over and over, about twenty times, as if she had hit overload and could not handle the new information. It was too much change for her to comprehend. Consequently, I did not invite her friends to eat with us this time.

Make sure you use their money for the most happiness they can have now. If they need or want something, get it for them. You do not want to feel guilty later. Of course, it would be foolish to let Mom have her diamond ring now.

21

Health/Doctors

Doctor's Visit

The caregiver or another adult needs to hear what the doctor says. Older people do not understand the medical results or prognosis, do not ask necessary questions, and cannot remember what the doctor said. Someone else needs to hear what the doctor said. With our access to the internet we can investigate illnesses online, better understand the options, and ask informed questions.

Relationship with Family Doctor

Fortunately, I went to high school with the man who has been Mom's doctor for many years now. He has been a **tremendous** help on numerous occasions.

Through the years I have sent him letters to document Mom's current status, like her more than 50 calls per year to the police, her seeing spots on the ceiling, and her locking herself in her upstairs bedroom when it got dark. (Actually, I learned later from her eye specialist that seeing spots on the ceiling can be a warning sign for macular degeneration.)

The doctor put Mom in the hospital when she received stitches in her head from a fall that occurred when her blood sugar was low.

I asked him to send her to an assisted living facility to recover which he did. He told me he could only keep her there for three weeks, and I told him that was all I needed. Mom was very social and was really lonely living by herself but would not admit it. Once she realized how wonderful it was to have people around and someone providing all her meals plus washing the dishes (which she always hated), she thought she would stay a few weeks. It was winter, and she would have been confined to her home since she no longer drove and was dependent on her elderly friends. She stayed there for four and a half years.

Introduce yourself to your parents' doctors. You will need their help. It might be in taking the drivers' licenses away, moving your parents to assisted living, assisting in moving them to another town with a new doctor, or discussing the end-of-life scenario.

The doctor warned me that Mom would soon need to leave the assisted living for more care in a skilled care facility. The assisted living probably kept her longer than normal because they needed the income. When she had the bleeding ulcer in the hospital and then could not walk, it was obviously the time to move her and probably made an easier transition for her.

Be an advocate for your parents and proactive with the doctors; insist on the right treatments factoring in their age, their will to live, and family genetics. Some doctors look on people in their 80s as "waiting to die." We know our family genes and whether we think our parents will live into their 90s. When my mother was bleeding to death at age 89, the surgeon told me he would not operate because of her age. I told him that I would not stand by and see my mother bleed to death. We agreed to decide in two days, and fortunately, she recovered by that time. Doctors consider the risk of surgery, best use of their energies, and insurance costs. You need to think about the "human factor": whether your parents would be strong enough to withstand surgery, their will to live, and their family genetic history.

Our parents treat doctors as gods, and usually do not question their decisions. Doctors are well educated and should be respected, but you have a right to question and understand medicines and treatments.

Keep a list of all your parents' medicines with their dosages, frequencies, and purpose. You will need this if there are questions from the pharmacy, insurance company, skilled care facility, or hospital, if they are admitted. Because of the side effects from medicine and the potential interactions between drugs, you want to minimize the number of drugs they take.

Keep the doctor informed of major changes you observe. You might see your parents across 24 hours while the doctor just sees them for a few minutes. As Mom showed more signs of dementia, periodically I sent the doctor a letter documenting Mom's changes in case I needed to force her to move to assisted living or gain Guardianship, which is complicated and might be expensive with lawyer and court fees.

My cousin initiated the formal court process to become his father's legal Guardian. I have not needed to do this because the Power of Attorney has resolved any of my situations.

Encourage physical therapy when needed. Staying active, strong, and mobile are important to aging parents. If your parents need therapy, and they can afford it, request the doctor to approve it. Have as much therapy as is recommended, and as your parents are willing to endure. After my mother's bleeding ulcer episode and her eight days being bedridden in the hospital, she had physical therapy to regain her mobility. This time it had little success, and she finally said it was too painful to continue. She has been in a wheelchair since. Her legs have atrophied and stay bent. She no longer can push her recliner completely back because her legs will not straighten, which means she must now sleep on her side. Her aides are pushing her recliner back some to gradually stretch those leg muscles.

Being in a wheelchair increases the risk for bedsores or boils, urinary tract infections, and poor circulation. Add this to incontinence and diabetes, and you have raw, sore skin. As Mom sits all the time in her wheelchair and is incontinent, she recently developed a boil on her bottom. My doctor friend told me about **Boudreaux's Butt Paste®. Get some for your parents if they are incontinent or in wheelchairs.** I found it at Walmart in the baby section. Desitin® Ointment for diaper rash might also be effective, but Mom was allergic to it. Changing positions or reclining some during the day may reduce pressure points. Bedsores can be a sign of nutritional deficiency.

If your parents are in wheelchairs, go to the specialty equipment store and see what custom cushions are available that fit in wheelchairs. Get the best available; your parent will sit on it most waking hours of the day. I wanted one with more support and cushioning effect. Some even have gel. Medicare paid for Mom's wheelchair, but I have purchased extra cushions. They need to be replaced periodically for various reasons. Boldly label all covers and foam pads with a permanent marker since the covers get washed.

I do ask the aides to transfer Mom to her recliner for several hours a day, so it provides a change for her sitting position and relieves the pressure points. The facility had a gel cushion they put in Mom's recliner to avoid bedsores or boils. The aides are very aware and try to avoid this issue.

There are alarms that can be attached to the person and connected to their wheelchair, so if your parents try to leave their wheelchairs, an alarm sounds. This is helpful for people who wander off. Mom does not need this.

The assisted living or skilled care facility will need scripts or prescriptions from the family doctor even for over-the-counter supplements including the Butt Paste®! This is another reason to have a good relationship with your parents' family doctor. Check with him or her before giving any supplements to your parents. I needed Mom's doctor to write up scripts for Citracal®, multivitamin, vitamin C, eye vitamin, glucosamine/chondroitin, baby aspirin, and Butt Paste®.

If your parents are diabetic, ask the doctor to check their feet with their shoes and socks off at each visit. Any wound or inflammation of the feet is a major concern because diabetics are slow to heal, especially in their feet. Mom has been hospitalized twice because she had foot infections that did not heal easily. One friend's father was diabetic and had a blister that did not heal for six months. Avoid cuts or wounds to their feet. I recommend custom fit shoes or orthotics, if they are diabetic. Medicare will help with this expense if the doctor writes a script.

Know the signs of stroke and what to do.

Signs of Stroke:

- Numbness
- Confusion
- Vision problems
- Dizziness
- Headaches
- Impaired speech
- Face drooping
- Inability to raise arms and keep both up
- The tongue pointing to one side when stuck out

Do not call the doctor, call 9-1-1, and get your parent to the hospital emergency room for evaluation. An immediate evaluation is critical for strokes. Strokes need to be treated by a doctor **within two hours** to minimize damage.

Mom had an incident when she was with me and could not make a complete sentence. She could say individual words but was unable to put them together for about fifteen minutes. I took her to ER, where the doctor did some tests like an EKG. He was not sure what caused it, but it might have been a TIA (transient ischemic attack), which is a mini-stroke, a temporary interruption of blood flow to part of the brain. These can be early signs of future strokes. Fortunately, Mom's speech recovered before we got to the hospital. Then I thought I had over-reacted, but the doctor said I did the right thing by having her checked.

Supplements

Consider these supplements to prevent problems.

Check with your family doctor before giving your parents any supplements.

Label any supplements you provide with your parents' names.

Doctors are trained to identify diseases, prescribe medicines, and perform surgery, but they are **not trained in nutrition and prevention of diseases**. There are several over-the-counter supplements that I felt were important for Mom's health since I take many of them myself. Be proactive in preventing problems. Below are some items to consider.

If parents are living in independent living and have increased dementia, do not allow them to take over-the-counter supplements at their own discretion. They can overdose themselves, or sometimes these items, such as cough medicine, can be strong and interfere with their regular medicines. You would not allow a two-year-old to take medicine, so remember they are becoming childlike.

- **Calcium with Vitamin D**: Mom was definitely getting shorter, so I asked for her to start taking a calcium supplement, such as Citracal®. It is important to avoid broken or brittle bones.

- **Glucosamine/Chondroitin**: Mom was having trouble walking and had pain in her knees. Arthritis and joint deterioration can impact seniors' mobility. I was already taking glucosamine/chondroitin and found it helpful for my knees. I asked for her to start taking this supplement, and it seemed to help. MSM (methylsulfonylmethane) can sometimes also reduce the pain of arthritis.

- **Another option for joints**: Joint Advantage Gold® by Dr. David Williams. Visit his website: www.drdavidwilliams.com

- **Eye Supplement:** Mom developed macular degeneration and was treated by an eye specialist, who told Mom to take this vitamin for her eyes, Ocuvite® PreserVision™ AREDS (for Age-Related Eye Disease Study) formula. My eye doctor suggested I take vitamins with lutein and zinc to reduce the risk of macular degeneration.

- **Aspirin:** After Mom had an event where she could not form sentences for about fifteen minutes, which might have been a mini-stroke or TIA (transient ischemic attack), the doctor suggested she take a daily aspirin. After taking a daily regular aspirin her skin started bruising very easily, so with the doctor's permission, I had the daily aspirin reduced to a low-dose, children's aspirin (81 mg).

- **Multivitamin**: Mom takes one daily multivitamin, such as Walmart's One Source Women's 50+.

- **Vitamin C**: This vitamin aids the immune system, so Mom takes one Vitamin C (500 mg) daily.

Neurologist

If your parents have memory or walking issues, schedule them with a neurologist. Your family doctor may need to refer them.

I knew Mom was having memory and walking problems. I took the initiative and made an appointment with a neurologist. When Mom realized where she was, she refused to go in. I went in and left her in the car. Eventually she agreed to go in because she did not want to be alone in the car. The neurologist asked, "What year is it?" Mom said, "Paula, tell the doctor what year it is!" Then he asked, "Who is the President?" Mom said, "Paula, tell him who the President is." He asked her to walk across the room. Mom turned to me and said, "Paula, get me up!" The doctor had the answers to his questions.

The neurologist looked at her hands, arms, and legs. Although she did not exhibit the distinctive tremors of Parkinson's disease in her hand and arm that my father (her husband) had, the doctor felt she had Parkinson's. There is no specific test for it. She no longer had fine motor skills in her hands, could barely write her name, could not put on jewelry or button blouses, and had difficulty in walking. She threw a fit saying she did not have Parkinson's and refused to go back to the doctor. This was difficult because doctors need to see a patient before they can renew a prescription. Fortunately, at my request, the family doctor, who saw Mom monthly, renewed the prescription.

My father was exposed to chemicals in World War II and as a blacksmith, and he worked near paints and other environmental concerns in the railroad shops. Mom might have been exposed by washing his contaminated clothing. The cause of Parkinson's disease is unknown although it can be hereditary. My father had signs of Parkinson's disease for about ten years before he died but did not exhibit any signs of dementia at his death at age 83.

Eye Specialist

Schedule yearly eye checkups for your parents.

Have their eyes checked for cataracts, glaucoma, blood vessel leakage, and macular degeneration. Diabetes can cause the blood vessels in the eyes to leak, which might require laser surgery.

With Mom's macular degeneration her regular eye doctor suggested she be treated by an eye specialist in my college town about 70 miles away. For many years my visits home were planned, so Mom could have regular trips to the eye specialist, who would give Mom shots in her eyes to retard the progress of macular degeneration. Once Mom was in the wheelchair, and I could not transfer her, I stopped these visits. Mom is still able to read the bingo card which has large numbers and to see her food with her good eye. You can tell one eye is worse because she has trouble with depth perception in eating her food. Of course, she will not admit it.

Podiatrist

As people age, they have trouble bending over to cut their toenails. Sometimes their toenails thicken or get fungus and are difficult to trim. Keep their toenails trimmed, so they do not get ingrown or infected. You might be able to cut their toenails or take them to a podiatrist. Initially they might fight you on this because of the cost. Once they go, they usually realize the need. Medicare covers some of the expense. I was trimming Mom's toenails recently, accidentally cut one too close, and made it bleed. This is a concern for diabetics.

Dentist

If your parents are eating less or have trouble chewing, have their teeth checked.

Your parents' dentures might have become uncomfortable or ill fitting. Weight loss or bone loss can affect the fit of their false teeth. Some foods, such as certain meats, fruits, and vegetables, are more difficult to chew and may be left out of their diet. Essential nutrients may be missed.

I noticed Mom was having trouble chewing her food, so I made an appointment with her dentist. Her bottom dentures were not fitting properly. He re-lined them which helped some. He told me that Mom was losing so much bone in her lower jaw that there was nothing else he could do.

Dementia and Parkinson's disease can affect seniors' swallowing which is a muscular action. Mom's caregivers now crush her pills as she is having trouble swallowing them.

Orthotics

Mom is diabetic and had several foot infections from poor choices in shoes; she chose style over function into her 80s! The family doctor wrote a script for her to purchase special shoes with a larger toe box. We went to a specialty store for orthotics to order them to fit her foot.

A portion of this expense was covered by Medicare. She wore high heels her whole adult life! She still tells me she wants some new black patent pumps! I should consider it now that she is in a wheelchair and does not have her weight on her feet.

Physical therapist

If your parents are hospitalized or off their feet for even a short period, they might need physical therapy. Their leg muscles atrophy quickly. The family doctor must prescribe this treatment, but you can request it or discuss it with him or her. I have requested it for Mom several times. Initially it energized her because she had one-on-one attention. The therapist even had Mom dancing around the room to increase her leg strength. It was beautiful! After she was hospitalized during the auction, she said it was too painful and did not want to continue it. For therapy to be effective, your parents must be willing to try.

22

Brief Summary of Dementia's Stages

Ask your doctor for complete descriptions or search online. (*See* **Help for Elders**.)

1. No problems

2. Very mild cognitive decline: forgets words, names, or keys, which is not obvious to others

3. Mild cognitive decline: has deficiencies in word-finding and decreased memory noticed by others

4. Moderate cognitive decline: has deficiencies in short term memory and decreased judgment and calculation, the ability to pay bills and handle finances

5. Moderately severe decline: has major memory gaps, such as day, date, or time, and needs help dressing

6. Severe decline: personality changes, anxiety, agitation, compulsive, repetitive actions, hallucinations, incontinence, long term memory problems, gets lost, and has difficulty conversing

7. Very severe decline: cannot make sentences, cannot walk,

has trouble swallowing, needs help with eating/toileting, and has frequent urinary tract infections and bedsores

Assess your parents' current stages of dementia.

Each might be at a different level. These might show up as a noticeable decline in learning, remembering, problem solving, and communicating.

23

Dementia

A person with dementia or Alzheimer's disease must have a personal advocate.

It is a matter of life and death. Without a personal advocate a person with Alzheimer's will have unmet needs and may even die because of oversights or honest mistakes.

The person with Alzheimer's will sadly be ignored, even when they share vital information or make an important request while an assertive personal advocate is less likely to be ignored and will take appropriate action if important requests are ignored at first.

I have definitely been an advocate for Mom on numerous occasions, especially when she had her bleeding ulcer.

When Mom was taken by ambulance from the assisted living to the hospital with what turned out to be a bleeding ulcer, the hospital was giving her blood transfusions to keep her alive. I had to advocate for a gastroenterologist to seek out the source of her blood loss.

When the endoscopy showed her stomach ulcer, and the doctor told me she was too old for surgical repair of the ulcer, I asked him if he had checked for the bacteria which is sometimes associated with stomach ulcers. He had not. But fortunately, he had taken a stomach biopsy which, upon checking, did indeed show the bacteria, and he prescribed the appropriate antibiotic to treat her ulcer.

Mom was very emotional about the 3-day auction of her cherished life possessions, which caused or aggravated her bleeding ulcer. Once I recognized her mental and emotional trauma from this event, I advocated for a sedative to be prescribed, so she could relax and heal in the hospital. The nurse understood, and this was accomplished. Happily, her ulcer healed by Monday, and I did not need to confront the doctor about surgery.

When Mom was released from the hospital to the new skilled care facility, I assumed they had transferred her prescription information, but that did not happen. I had to personally contact the hospital doctor and get him to re-issue prescriptions for her medications, including the antibiotic treatment for her ulcer.

When Mom was moved to the second skilled care facility a month later, the prescription information transfer was missed again. I took all her medicines to the pharmacy and had the pills checked, counted, and re-labeled for acceptance by the new facility. The pharmacy did not charge me for their efforts since Mom was a long term client, which saved buying all new medicine.

Mom loves to eat. Whenever she and her tablemates complained about the food, I personally joined her for many meals, and initially advocated to the kitchen manager for more nutritious and appetizing food. I gave her several months to take corrective action. When I was not satisfied, I sent a letter to the Board of Directors.

Dementia is called "the long good-bye" because your parents slowly lose their memory over the course of years. You must pace yourself for the long haul and not burn out in the early phases. Watch for signs of fatigue and depression in yourself. Treat yourself to fun trips with your friends and walks with the dog as healthy diversions. Realize that it is emotionally painful to slowly lose the parents you knew.

The stage or level of dementia is one indicator when your parents should be moved out of their home. With people living longer, this issue is growing. When their dementia is obvious to their friends, it is probably time to get help or consider moving them. My dear friend sent me a list of the dementia stages she received at a support meeting. When I recognized how advanced Mom was on the dementia scale, it forced me to realize she needed to move to assisted living primarily for her own safety. Unfortunately, diseases such as dementia and Alzheimer's make dealing with your parents exponentially more difficult because they are losing their reasoning ability.

A cousin who volunteers with dementia associations offered these comments:

"It's good that you are researching dementia. It's helpful to understand what's happening to Catherine's brain and her perception of the world. She's not 'being difficult' or 'uncooperative' or whatever; in fact *she's doing the best she can with what's left.* It's sad for her and for you, too. But it's good to *understand* and make the best of the 'hand she is dealt today.'

"One of the last portions of the brain to go involves our earliest memories. *Early musical memories are among the last things to go....* Music can trigger a 'good day' for him or her. Good care for patients with dementia will include music therapy, including sing-alongs."

There is a high probability your parents will gradually lose their short-term memory due to dementia. Easy test questions to ask are:

>> What year is it?

>> Who is President of the U.S.?

Sometimes people do not want to see the aging changes and avoid them. As a young adult, I did not want to see Grandpa with dementia which, then, was called hardening of the arteries. I wanted to remember him as the vibrant, handsome, funny, strong man I knew. My parents feared for Grandma's well-being and moved him to a nursing home close to their home. Grandma was worn down, and Grandpa did not always recognize her. Mom took Grandma almost every day to feed Grandpa his supper for the three years he lived there. It was a living hell for him because he constantly wanted to go to his childhood home. He was extremely strong and fought the aides, who had to tie him down. As a mature adult, I realize we must face our duties and responsibilities even though they are difficult at times.

Consider joining a support group:

- Learn what worked for others.
- Get guidelines and educational materials.
- Share your emotions and feelings.
- Others are dealing with the same issue – you are not alone.

Mom and most of her friends played bridge for almost 70 years, and I think that mental stimulation helped keep their minds sharp. Mom played the piano for many years; another friend still plays the piano at 91, which stimulates activity in multiple sections of the brain.

Mom thought it was a sin to sweat, so she did not exercise much. Her two brothers were very active with walking and bike riding. All three developed various levels of dementia in their late 80s. Mom is the only one of the three who developed adult onset diabetes, which she attributed to taking prednisone for several weeks to treat an allergic reaction to another drug. Her being significantly overweight at that time might have contributed; her brothers were not overweight.

Several articles mention that diabetes increases your risk of getting dementia.

Sometimes dementia affects the frontal portion of the brain which controls judgment. These people no longer have a filter on what they say and do. This is why some people curse or say hurtful words, and their behavior changes. Good manners might be lost.

People with dementia might exhibit these types of symptoms:

- Paranoia or anxiety
- Memory loss
- Poor judgment
- Faulty reasoning or trouble with abstract thinking
- No sense of time and place
- Problems with walking and balance
- Loss of communication skills
- Neglect of personal care and safety
- Inappropriate behavior
- Repeat the same questions
- Become lost or disoriented in familiar places
- Cannot follow directions
- Do not recognize and are confused about familiar people
- Have trouble with calculations and routine tasks, such as paying the bills

You will realize when it is time to stop asking your parents about recent events. As their dementia increases, anything they tell you will not be accurate, and you do not want to make them uncomfortable. Mom cannot remember what she had for supper, but she can remember something fun or significant, like attending a church meeting or winning at bingo. I limit my questions to Mom about whether her last meal was good. I do not ask my uncle any questions to avoid making him uncomfortable. Mom has difficulty with the day of the week and time of day. Realize your parents may argue with you about these things and avoid confrontations, if possible. Their reasoning ability is probably lost. When I am with Mom or my uncle, I just tell them about my activities; I don't expect them to contribute much to the conversation.

DEMENTIA

These symptoms show the progression of Mom's dementia:

Mom saw spots on the ceiling. This could be a warning sign of macular degeneration.

Mom was paranoid about people trying to break into her home and called the police over 50 times in one year. She "saw" people watching her house. She had the signs of "Sundowner's Syndrome" and became fearful at night.

Her vision was declining due to macular degeneration.

She was cooking less. Her blood sugar level got out of balance.

These were warnings she needed to move to assisted living.

She repeated what she said two to five times in a short period. Some people stopped conversing with her in the assisted living.

She was no longer able to pay her bills.

She does not know what year it is, or who is President.

She cannot remember what she had for supper (short-term memory issues).

Mom started wiping her nose, mouth, and hands repetitively as someone would with an obsession.

Her handwriting declined.

She does not know the day of the week or time of day.

She became incontinent.

She was unable to shower alone (loss of mobility) and dress herself (loss of fine motor skills).

When Mom could no longer walk and was in a wheelchair, I moved her to a skilled care facility at the doctor's direction.

It was sad when she forgot my birthday last year, but she remembered it a few days late this year!

She stopped watching TV (vision or memory issue).

She cannot remember how to put on her bra; many times her breasts are hanging down below the bra! She still insists on wearing one.

In the last few months she has had trouble remembering her husband of 54 years (long-term memory issues).

These issues are common for wheelchair patients with their reduced mobility:

- She developed a boil, which is a major concern, because she is diabetic.
- She is having repetitive urinary tract infections.

In the past few months Mom started having trouble swallowing her pills, so the facility is crushing them for her. The facility initiated this change.

She is sleeping more during the day. She nodded off when I had her in the car. She is napping at the meal table waiting for her food or in the lobby when I come to see her. She is alert while I am talking to her.

A few weeks ago **she called 9-1-1; this really upset the nursing home** because the police came to investigate. The phone company told me that I cannot block 9-1-1 from her phone. The facility wanted me to block all outgoing calls from her phone. Then she would not be able to call me, so I would not allow that. I do not know if she was afraid or dialed it by accident trying to call me since my area code starts with "9-1". I hope it does not happen again!

Last month we ate in a room across the hall from her room; she could not figure out where we were. She could not understand why I brought in food and asked the same four or five questions about twenty times.

On the phone she told me there were two men in her room, and one "put his penis up my ass." Immediately I called the nurses' station to investigate; fortunately, one of my favorite nurses was on duty. She did not have an incident report; they do have male nurses at this facility. I had just read an article about sexual abuse in nursing homes! Upon further investigation the nurse called back to tell me the male nurse inserted a suppository! So keep an open mind and your sense of humor!

Recently she was incoherent and managed to slide out near the foot of the bed even with the two guard rails. Thankfully, she did not break any bones. The nurses thought she could have a urinary tract infection, sent a urine sample for testing, and got an antibiotic prescription from the doctor. A few days later she was calling my name and thought I was visiting there. They had me talk to her on the phone to assure her I was in North Carolina. The nurse thought Mom was having a reaction to the antibiotic. They notified the doctor; he changed the antibiotic, and Mom calmed down. I feel the nurses at this facility take excellent care of Mom.

Sometimes she is having difficulty finding the words she wants to say.

She does remember when she plays bingo and wins!

Fortunately, she still knows my cousin and me and recognizes our voices. In the past she would talk for over ten minutes per call, but now the calls are only a few minutes as she has trouble remembering anything to tell me.

Mom has four friends in her facility, but no longer visits with them, and has trouble with more than a few minutes of conversation.

The nurse called to say Mom slid out of her wheelchair on the floor and scraped her back. I talked to Mom, who said her back hurt, but she was okay. The nurse did not think she broke anything. The aide put her nightgown on and saw another woman who was not supposed to be walking by herself. When she left Mom alone, Mom fell out of her chair. Of course, you must consider neglect or abuse, but I could tell by the nurse's voice that she was upset about the incident. These types of accidents are going to happen.

This week the skilled care facility requested that I decrease Mom's bed to just one bedrail. The state inspector does not want people confined and believes there is more danger when a person climbs over the bedrail. I told the facility that Mom requires two bedrails, and they have my signed form authorizing this. Mom does not remember that she cannot walk and support any of her own weight. I certainly do not want her getting out of bed in the middle of the night by herself and falling. The facility called again to insist on just one bedrail; I refused. Mom is not aggressive or agile enough to go over the bedrail. Knowing her as well as I do, she is the safest with two bedrails.

My Thoughts

In dealing with parents with dementia:

- **Do not argue.** This is futile and a waste of energy.
- **Do not try to use reason or logic.**

They no longer have this capability. Distracting them or changing the subject usually works to stop their arguing or insisting about an erroneous fact, such as Grandma died four weeks ago. I could not convince her there was no man outside watching her house; I could only distract her.

Mom seems to have grown more demanding and self-centered. Maybe this is related to her returning to that child-like state.

Mom was well into Stage 4 when she moved to assisted living. When I moved her into a skilled care facility, she was in Stage 6 and had a few items in Stage 7 (cannot walk and needs help with toileting).

As I write this, I realize Mom has more signs of the **final** stage of dementia. In the last few months she is not swallowing her pills, which they are now crushing. I thought it could be related to her Parkinson's disease, but Stage 7 dementia lists inability to swallow. She was not coherent the other night and managed to get out of bed even with the rails and slid to the floor. It turns out that she has a urinary tract infection, and frequent infections are also listed in Stage 7 along with bedsores and boils. The nurse said they started her on seven days of antibiotics but will keep her on a half dose of antibiotics forever. The director has moved Mom to a different meal table which has an aide nearby to help feed people, so she can help Mom when needed.

Another thing was so different when I was there recently. I brought in KFC one night because she loves fried chicken, mashed potatoes, and cole slaw. We sat in a private room with a small table, but she could not handle even this small amount of change. She did not know where she was although she was across the hall from her own room. She kept asking me over and over, like a tape playing, maybe twenty times – Why did I buy food when she had food. What is the food? Where did I get it? Why did I bring it in? Where are we? At that point I knew she could not handle bringing in her friends any more for a meal.

Mom still remembers how painful my birth was. She still remembers Daddy's suicide. She knows I had her sale and compiled the book of Daddy's letters in her honor. She knows I was there recently. For her, any financial transactions are clear, and she still remembers events with powerful emotions.

It was terribly upsetting when I realized she is exhibiting symptoms of Stage 7 because that means death is looming closer. No matter how prepared we think we are for our parents' deaths, we are not.

24

Cleaning Out Houses

Tie brightly colored ribbon to anything you want to keep. Each sibling can use a different color.

I had Mom's auction before I moved items I wanted to my home as I needed to be home to meet the moving van. To identify to the auction team each item I wanted to keep, I securely attached bright ribbon to it. This seemed to work well. If they accidentally brought an item out for the auction, it was easy to catch.

Keep anything you think you want. You can get rid of it later if you change your mind. Once it is gone, you cannot get it back! There were only a couple of items that I wish I had kept. There was only one item, a walnut chest, I bought out of the auction because it was going for $75. Overall, I probably kept too much! Since it was on multiple floors, I did not realize the volume until it got to my house!

I felt overwhelmed in cleaning out Mom's house. It took so much work to go through my parents' lifetime accumulation in their 4,000 sq. foot house and basement.

With regard to emptying your parents' home, think about what approach you plan to take. People have many different techniques. You need to decide what is right for you and your siblings. Only you know what is important.

- You might want to make a list of the things you want and start taking them now if your parents will permit this. They still own it until they give it to you. Mom did not give me anything until I insisted on the auction. Then she told me I could have whatever I wanted.

- Clean out the basement, attic, and guest rooms before they move.

- One friend just took one weekend to collect the wanted items then turned everything in the parents' house over to an auctioneer.

- Two cousins did not go through anything; they sold the house and contents. My other cousin and I wish we had known; we would have gone through the family pictures and bought the family keepsakes. I realize now why their mother so wisely gave me several family pictures and pieces of flow blue china many years earlier! She knew her children had no sentimental attachments to anything.

- There were many family keepsakes and treasures that I wanted. I found many wonderful surprises. I read the over 200 sympathy cards Mom received when Daddy died. I found my father's almost 700 World War II letters that were priceless. I found the 16mm film of me at ages 2 to 4 with my parents, grandparents, neighbors, and friends. I found letters from my grandfather's trip to Panama, where he worked when the canal was built. I found letters from my great-grandfather to his future bride about their wedding plans. I took years to sort through **everything**. This is my family history. I do not know if it was worth all the time I have invested in my parents' stuff, but I felt the need to personally review everything.

- My cousins and I also had to clean out our grandparents' house. Our old bachelor uncle had lived there for almost twenty years after our grandparents died, and by that time our parents were not able to clean it out. I did find treasures there, too.

At Grandma's house we sorted everything into four categories:

- Family treasures (such as pictures) or things we wanted to keep
- Clothing to Salvation Army or Goodwill – first go through every pocket and purse!
- Trash to the alley – the trash collectors were wonderful!
- Items for the auction – we sold everything that was left!

I had used this same scheme for cleaning out Mom's house, but I had very little trash there. Mom had some vintage clothing and hats that I kept in the auction. Each person has to decide what is right for them.

Consider selling those unique, valuable items online. With the success of e-Bay some items might bring more money by selling them online instead of a local auction. I knew many of Mom's items were fragile; it would cost money to move them to my town and would require more time.

Many Depression-era parents have accumulated lots of stuff that will require sorting. Their generation grew up very needy, so their belongings were precious to them. They also recycled and reused long before it became "fashionable," so they kept everything.

People collect everything, so limit what you throw away. I threw away very little at Mom's house. We even sold the empty coffee cans (you cannot get those any more), hangers, hats, and cardboard jewelry boxes. Most of the clothes I took to Goodwill or Salvation Army. If you have questions, ask an Estate Sale team or an auctioneer or check online.

The belongings need to be sorted and disposed of before you can successfully sell the house or put it on the market. People need to be able to visualize their belongings in the house. Also, Mom had many valuables that might disappear if I allowed strangers in the house before the sale.

What are your parents' wishes for the house? Does a sibling want it? Have they been the primary caregivers? Should they get the house at a reduced price for their efforts?

Realize that you might need to do repairs to your parents' home because they probably did not perform any maintenance in the last ten or fifteen years. One friend repaired the basement foundation and replaced windows, siding, and gutters. Another friend pulled up old carpeting to expose hardwood flooring. One friend is selling her mother's home "as is" since it is structurally sound, but people are complaining that it is "dated." You will have to weigh the cost, time, and efforts of updating the house versus selling it "as is." Can you select colors, materials, and fabrics that will satisfy all potential buyers? What is the return on your time and expense?

Once the house has been emptied, you can auction it, sell it yourself, or list it with a real estate agent. I have been trying to sell Mom's house as "for sale by owner" but have not been successful yet. Total the tax bill, yard maintenance, utility bills, insurance, etc., so you know the true cost of holding the house. Hopefully the price of real estate will increase soon.

25

Dividing the Belongings

Consider a mediator in dealing with the siblings if there are major problems dividing the belongings.

As an only child this was not an issue for me. Being an only child has its pluses and minuses. You make all the decisions, get the inheritance – hopefully some remains as your reward for your good care for them – but it also means you do all the work!

Beware that money can change people. Siblings and their spouses might have different values or wishes than you do. Do the right thing to have a clear conscience.

One neighbor woman had five sisters. They put numbers one through six in a hat. Each person drew a number. Starting with number one through number six each person got to select one thing they wanted, and this continued until they did not want anything else. There were no values assigned to anything. Sets of silverware and dishes were considered one item. This was a very friendly and successful approach.

Sometimes dollar values are assigned to everything. Each sibling is given a total value they can select, but this requires the expense of an unbiased third party to appraise everything.

Regarding my grandparents' house, my cousins and I took what we wanted. Fortunately, there were no issues over who got what. The rest was sold in an auction along with the house.

Mom did not tell me to give anything to anybody. She told me I could have whatever I wanted. Some people were dear family friends, who would like a keepsake from Mom. Whenever I found something that I knew a close friend or relative would appreciate, I gave or mailed it to them. My cousin's daughter wanted our Grandmother's antique cedar chest. One close friend's daughter collects roosters, so I sent her a brass rooster as a reminder of Mom. One friend collects aprons, so I sent her a couple. Another close friend collects pink depression glass, so I gave her a casserole. Another friend decorates for holidays, so I gave her a china Easter egg. People really seemed to appreciate a keepsake memory from Mom. It kept my mind off self-pity by thinking about giving pleasure to other people. Mom would have made more money if I sold these things, but seeing friends' faces receiving the gifts gave me motivation to continue.

26

Risks and Choices

I knew the auction of Mom's belongings might cause a stroke or even kill her. Because she was raised during the Depression, her belongings were her identify. Even though she had been in an assisted living for four and a half years, unable to return to her house for months, and not able to use the beautiful things in her house, she was not ready to let them go! That is why the sale almost killed her. I had already moved the items she selected and I could fit into her room at the assisted living. The day before the auction she almost died with a seizure and was moved to the hospital's intensive care with a bleeding ulcer. I had to have the nurse sedate her to get through the weekend. They gave her six pints of blood in three days. After that she never regained her ability to walk and has been in a wheelchair.

From my perspective, I knew she would never return home and enjoy her beautiful things again. I had not rushed the auction by waiting four and a half years. I felt in limbo because I could not return to work knowing I was responsible for having the auction and selling the house. By the time I had the auction it was mid-July and 98 degrees. It turned out to be a three-day auction! I also knew the house would never sell while it was **full**.

Realize there are risks involved with major decisions regarding your parents. Weigh the risks, make the decision, and deal with the consequences.

When I visited Mom last month I felt her suppers were not acceptable, made notes, and collected comments from other residents. Recently Mom was very upset two times in one week about her poor suppers and told me she was hungry. She stated, "I might need to move!" My mother rarely complains about the facility. That prompted me to send a complaint letter. The Administrator replied they took an informal survey, and over 80% gave favorable comments. They offered me the opportunity to move my mother to a facility that might better satisfy her appetite. This could force my decision to move Mom to my town. I will investigate my options because I certainly don't want Mom hungry and unhappy.

27

Discussions with Parents

Some parents will not be willing to discuss death and wills, but it is important, so you can execute their wishes. You need to discuss this while they have a clear mind. Several times I tried to discuss these things with Mom, but she was unwilling to think about death.

These are topics to discuss with your parents:

- When one parent dies, where will the remaining parent want to live? This might change later, but it is good to have the discussion now without grief entering the conversation.

- Insurance. Ask about all types of insurance (accident, medical, prescription, life, term, car, house, umbrella, and long-term care) including account numbers, contacts, and addresses.

- Wills/disbursement of their assets and belongings. Does the will need to be updated? Are there any special requests not included in the will?

   I asked Mom if she wanted to give anything away. She said, "No, but you can have anything you want." That was wonderful news since she had some beautiful things. She even paid to have the items I kept moved to my house!

- Funeral arrangements or plans. Do your parents have pre-paid plans at a specific funeral home? Is there a funeral home they prefer? Is there a minister they prefer? What special songs or singer should be included? Who would need to be notified? Ask them to select their caskets.

Two years ago my uncle's basic funeral in a small Midwest town cost over $5,000 without the cemetery plot or grave marker. My father's funeral cost $8,000 sixteen years ago. If there is a more expensive casket, vault, and extra limousines, a funeral can be over $10,000.

If money is tight and your parents are close to needing Medicaid, it is important to use their money to pay for their funeral before it is all gone. Someone will have to pay for their funeral, so consider pre-paying for a funeral now.

- Obituary. Ask them to write their life's accomplishments. If they are not willing, write the information and ask them to review it. Write it now, so you will not forget important items in your grief and rush. I wrote Mom's obituary and read it to her. She did not like it, so she changed it! I was making progress.

- Eulogy. Will you or someone give a eulogy at the funerals? Think about it and make notes. I knew I would be too upset at my father's funeral to give the eulogy, so my son offered to read it. At my uncle's funeral I had the minister read what I wrote. He did not know my uncle, so this was very helpful.

- Burial plots and headstones. Do they want to be cremated? Where do they want their ashes? Do they own burial plots? If not, where do they want to be buried? Are they entitled to be buried in a military cemetery, and is that their wishes? Ask them to select and purchase these plots now. Ask them to select their headstones, which can be personalized and installed on the plots now with their names and birth dates. The death date can be added later. If they do not select what they want now, they are at your mercy. Mom has her burial plot, but I could not get her to select her headstone.

To personalize their headstones:

- If your parents are Christian, consider adding a cross.

- If your mother is a member of DAR, consider adding the DAR emblem as a separate stone.

- If your father is a Mason, consider adding a Masonic emblem.

- Since my father worked for the railroad for 45 years, I plan to put a train on his, which will be a joint headstone with Mom.

- Veteran. If your loved one was a veteran, do you plan to have a military style funeral with the gun salute and the flag draped coffin?

  Either way, have the funeral home notify the Veterans Administration to order a nice plaque for the grave with their name, rank, branch of service, birth date, and death date. My father's has: CSF (Chief Ship Fitter, a Chief Petty Officer) Paul L. Edwards, US Navy, World War II, Birth (Month, Day, Year) – Death (Month, Day, Year). I like that his includes "World War II"; my uncle's does not have that although he served then, too.

- Mason. If your loved one was a Mason, he should be buried wearing his Masonic apron.

28

Role Reversal —
You Are the Parent Now!

At some point you take on the role of parent, and the parent becomes the child. You must make the decisions and do the right thing in the right way. Always look for better ways of doing things.

We reached the point where Mom was not paying her bills on a regular basis or paying them twice. Someone at the assisted living was writing and mailing the checks, but Mom would take her bills and tell her what to do. She was 88 when I told her I was paying her bills. She was really angry with me for meddling in her affairs, but I knew it was time for me to take this responsibility. She was losing control of her life and losing her sense of accomplishment and purpose, and she did not like it! She was terribly mad at me because paying her bills was her only job or meaningful monthly contribution. Now there was nothing for her to do. This was the point when I realized that now I am the parent, and she is the child.

Now you are in control, and they are losing control. Your parents will not want to easily give up control of their lives. Their decision making becomes cloudy or non-existent because, with dementia, the judgment portion of the brain is affected first. At some point you must take control of their lives and make the decisions. This can be an emotional roller coaster if you have a parent like mine. I had never given her any indication of being money hungry, but Mom really fought me on taking control of her finances.

At this point you simply do what you know to be the right thing and do it right. You no longer ask them for permission. You take charge, make decisions, and move forward. It will be much easier for you once you get to this frame of mind and accept this role. Your parents will still not like your taking control, but it is necessary. They will gradually stop fighting you when they see your good choices and trust your actions. They won't have the motivation or energy to do the work themselves.

Aging causes the person to become more childlike in many ways. It is like dealing with a two-year-old, but you can pick up a two-year-old or put the child in time out. Neither of these options accomplishes the desired results with an aging parent.

Mom would throw temper tantrums if she did not get her way or what she wanted. You have to select her clothes and dress her. She lets you know if she does not like a food by spitting it out. You need to cut her meat, tell her what the foods are, and sometimes help her eat like a two-year-old.

She gradually required daily use of Depends, adult diapers, and became incontinent like a young child. My cousin says we start out helpless in diapers and years later revert to helpless in diapers.

She cannot reason or be logical, so I am not able to explain my rationale for decisions.

Recently she demanded I put on her lipstick, comb her hair, put on her jewelry, put on a sweater, wipe her hands, dry her hands, and take her to the dining room. One friend who was a school teacher and dealt with an aging mother says children start out as ego-centric, and, as people age, they become ego-centric again.

Many times Mom refused to go to the bathroom when asked. I had her out of town to an eye specialist and knew we had over an hour drive. I asked her to go to the bathroom before we left, and she refused to try. The nurses could hear our loud disagreement and understood my position. Of course thirty minutes down the road she had to go to the bathroom while on the highway. It was torture and comical having her trying to use a plastic pan in the car! Have a potty, bag, and paper towels handy just like you did for your two-year-old!

29

Change in Perspective

In recent years Mom is less critical and has changed her viewpoint. She never wanted to go through everything in her house and do that large amount of work to have her sale; I did. I compiled Daddy's almost 700 letters to her into a book. She never considered undertaking this enormous, time-consuming job; I did. I continue to take care of her house which has not sold. She realizes that I have done and continue to do a tremendous amount of work for her. I buy her clothes and jewelry because she still cares about her appearance and sets a good example for others. People compliment her on how nice she looks! Now her attitude has changed to appreciation. She thanks me for everything I do! She now thanks the people at her facility for helping her. This is truly a blessing!

30

Desired End Result

Galatians 6:9 *And let us not grow weary in well-doing, for in due season we shall reap, if we do not lose heart.*

My friends and I say, **"Finish well."**

You do not want to live with regret or guilt.

Use their money for their happiness while they are alive.

Do whatever you can to make them feel special. Tell them whatever is true:

- They are good people and helped others.
- They had a worthy life, and their life mattered. You would not be here if it was not for them!
- They were great parents. If you feel the need to take care of them and read this, they must have done a good job raising you!
- They are going to heaven – if they are Christians.
- You love them.

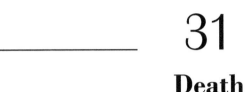

31

Death

When death is near:

- Have their minister or yours visit with them and you.
- Have Hospice notified.

Help your parents be at peace.

Ask them if there is anyone they need to forgive or ask for forgiveness to give them peace.

"Forgive and give as if it were your last opportunity. Love like there's no tomorrow, and if tomorrow comes, love again." by Max Lucado

If your parents are Christians, convince them they are going to heaven.

Ask them to repeat after you: "Lord Jesus, I repent of my sins, come into my heart, I make you my Lord and Savior. I ask all these things through your son, Jesus Christ. Amen." Mom repeated this for my benefit recently.

Mom has been a Christian her whole life and attended church, but at this time she is not at peace with dying. She has accepted Jesus as her Lord and Savior and repented for her sins. She believes her parents are in heaven. When I ask her if she is going to heaven, she says, "I don't know." It seems to be an issue of being worthy although Christianity is based on faith, grace, and Christ's resurrection to forgive our sins. I do not think anyone validated her in her youth. I continue to tell her what a good mother she was, and that I love her. I want Mom to be at peace with dying; it is a fact of life that happens to everyone.

What a blessing that one grandmother died in bed in her own house at 94. My other grandmother lived in her own house until she was 95, went to the hospital for two days, and died. Neither one had dementia nor suffered. Both of them had an adult child living with them. Everyone is not that fortunate.

At some point you will be in charge of your parents' lives.

It is important you understand their wishes concerning end of life. You might have to decide if you put in a feeding tube or pull the plug on life support. It is difficult deciding how long people should live. Does all the technology keep people alive beyond when their lives are meaningful?

Mom's older brother, a bachelor, had lived in a skilled care facility for about four years and was confined to a wheelchair and had dementia. He had a severe heart attack and was sent to the hospital. I happened to be in my hometown; my cousin called me from Illinois after six AM and asked me to go to the hospital. Tom's doctor was already there. He said, "You know Tom is 92 and has a do not resuscitate order." I replied, "I understand and agree." I could tell Tom was in severe pain by his movements, so I requested the doctor keep him out of pain. The doctor ordered him morphine. I called my cousin to tell her how serious it was. She notified her two siblings and started the six hour drive to our hometown. I stayed with Tom and tried to comfort him. After lunch I brought Mom to say good-bye to her brother. My three cousins arrived with their dad, the younger brother. We all had an opportunity to tell Tom we loved him, we didn't want him to suffer, and we let him go. We left several hours later to take our parents home and get some supper. We all four arrived at the hospital about seven

PM, but Tom died a few minutes before we returned. I intended to spend the night at the hospital and be with Tom when he died. He was a very private person, and maybe that was the way he wanted it.Maybe he didn't know we would return. It is very sad to have a family member die regardless of their age and circumstance. I wrote his eulogy and attended his funeral; I requested Mom and her younger brother's minister preach his funeral. I eventually helped my cousin clean out his belongings. I found a few ways to honor Tom in death.

Mom would never have this discussion about death. Maybe she wanted to die when her possessions were sold. Maybe I should have let her die when she had the seizure in the hospital. I did not want my mother to bleed to death. I selfishly did not believe I could handle the 3-day auction plus her funeral. I would not change my choice at that point in time. Since then she has been in a wheelchair, which almost confines her to the facility, and now her dementia and her quality of life are much worse. If I have another deciding point, I have to let her go. I believe studying dementia and writing this book were to help me reach this major decision.

I was in shock when Daddy shot and killed himself. That was his choice when the quality of his life was significantly declining with his Parkinson's disease and back pain.

He was diagnosed with Parkinson's disease about 1986. Due to this disease combined with his sleep apnea he had a permanent tracheotomy, which he said was the worst thing that ever happened to him. He loved people so much, but he had difficulty talking when his sinus drainage would clog his "trach." Plus he was starting to fall more often. The Parkinson's had stolen his facial expressions and his big smile that would light up a room. It was a living hell.

Daddy had always been so active, independent, and adventuresome — a "goer" and a "doer." He had always been a "take charge" type person. I think it was difficult for him to accept his future in a wheelchair. He had bad back pains that the doctors could not relieve. There was a seven year difference in my parents' age. It was never a problem until Daddy was about 82, and Mom was 75. He wanted to stay home; she still wanted to go and do. He found peace and comfort in his own way. The more I see of aging, I better understand his loving choice to not be a burden on Mom as his Parkinson's progressively got worse. After much thought, I considered his choice to be a courageous, loving act.

One family friend said so astutely at his funeral, "Your mom is not the nurse type." He was right. Daddy married her for many wonderful traits, but that was not one he considered in his 20s. Not everyone can handle that role. I knew I could not be the sole caregiver for Mom. Recognize your own strengths and limitations.

In many ways I feel I am honoring Daddy by taking care of Mom's needs. He took care of her for 54 years, and now it has been my turn for almost sixteen years.

The elderly do commit suicide. Do what you can to prevent it. Suicide is a shock and a waste of a life. Parkinson's disease, dementia, depression, and loneliness can contribute to this possibility. Remove ammunition and potential weapons. Watch for any signs that indicate they are thinking about it. Daddy asked me if my son wanted a piece of his luggage. In hindsight that was a clue that he was considering suicide because he was giving away his belongings.

One person I know tried to commit suicide and was unsuccessful. It just made things worse because it created more health problems.

I knew when I had to finally put my 17-year-old dog to sleep, but that is not socially acceptable for humans.

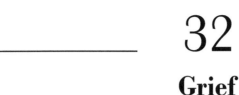

32

Grief

Hospice can offer guidance and support for dealing with death.

Your minister can offer consolation from grief.

It is difficult when your parents die. It is hard to accept you are now the older generation. One friend felt lost after her parents' deaths. Another felt adrift; a third friend felt a void. You instantly become an orphan.

You do not want your parents to suffer, but you do not want them to die. You want to be done with the work and responsibility, but you do not want to lose them. They told you they loved you, treated you special, and gave you gifts. You do not want to lose that unique connection or bond. There are many mixed feelings.

Do what needs to be done. Do the best you can now, so you avoid feeling guilty at their deaths.

Mom thinks her parents died a few months ago, and her brother did not take her to their funeral. She is grieving for them now, but they died over twenty years ago, and she wants her inheritance! Actually she attended their funerals and received her fair portion of their money. I tried to comfort her by saying they died twenty years ago, but she does not understand the timeframe or logic. All I could finally say was, "I'm sorry." She is going through the grieving process again, and I cannot prevent it.

Dementia is, as I said, the "long good-bye." In many ways it is sad. I miss my real mother. I have started the grieving process over Mom in the last year or so since her mind and personality disappeared. With her amazing memory gone she is no longer the mother I knew. She was the life of the party, excellent at telling jokes and making people laugh. She was a good cook and bridge player. Now she barely remembers her husband, her previous life, or her family history although she still wants to wear nice clothes and pretty jewelry. She knows I do things for her and handle her business. She still wants to know anything involved with her money. It is wonderful she remembers my son, a cousin, and me.

Mom talked non-stop for 90 years. Sometimes I wanted to hit a "stop" button! Now she does not have much to say, cannot remember what she had for supper, or what she did during the day. How I miss my mother, and she is still here.

You will feel a major loss when your parent dies. I have accepted Daddy's death, but I had a hole in my heart for many years. I still miss Daddy after sixteen years! Visiting his grave seems to give me some connection with him. Compiling his World War II letters into a book helped me feel closer to him, paid tribute to his accomplishments, and emphasized his values. That closeness and effort to honor him helped heal my loss.

One friend said about a year after the death of her 96-year-old father, who was always vivacious and full of life, "This has been difficult for me, as I continue to grieve for my father every day. He is still a constant memory to me. What a stronghold he has, even in death, as he did in life."

These are five steps to healing, and everyone seems to go through most of the steps at their own pace. These may all occur in this sequence, only one or two may happen, or the order may be changed.

However, it is good to be aware that these feelings may exist, so you can work through them.

Grief from www.wikipedia.com:

"The 5 stages are:

1. Denial

2. Anger

3. Bargaining

4. Depression

5. Acceptance

"Although the death of a spouse may be an expected change, it is a particularly powerful loss of a loved one. A spouse often becomes part of the other in a unique way: many widows and widowers describe losing 'half' of themselves. After a long marriage, at older ages, the elderly may find it a very difficult assimilation to begin anew.

"When an adult child loses a parent in later adulthood it is considered 'timely' and a normative life course event. This allows the adult children to feel a permitted level of grief. Research demonstrates that the death of a parent in midlife is not a normative event by any measure, but a major life transition. Depending on the individual this transition can impact the child's life in many different ways. The child may evaluate their own life more closely or look into their own mortality. Others may shut out friends and family while trying to process losing someone they have had the longest relationship with.

"An adult may be expected to cope with the death of a parent in a less emotional way; however, it can still invoke extremely powerful emotions. This is especially true when the death occurs at an important or difficult period of life, such as when becoming a parent, graduation or other times of emotional stress. It is important to recognize the effects that the loss of a parent can cause and address these. As an adult, the willingness to be open to grief is often diminished. A failure to accept and deal with loss will only result in further pain and suffering."

Aging, death, grief, and loss are all parts of the natural order of life. Strong and mixed feeling are a part of this grieving process. Often the remaining person feels sorry for himself/herself along with the strong loss. Sometimes these emotions may be seen in physical symptoms, such as depression or extreme anxiety. The person may be hesitant to make the simplest of decisions. Instead of "bargaining" mentioned above, some people have a numbness or lack of feeling. The widow may become obsessive about keeping fanatically busy. It is important to acknowledge these feelings, let them out, and not keep them bottled up inside.

Women live longer than men. Women should not underestimate themselves. They possess an amazing ability to adapt and respond to new situations.

People grieve because they fear the unknown. They are not sure what happened. People feel guilty for things they did not do for the person before he or she died. They were not done, and it is time to move on in life. Perhaps it can be a helpful reminder to do more for those we love who are alive.

Another reason people grieve is related to the insecurity of our lives. One day our life is orderly, and the next day it is chaos. Following death, there is often much disorder, and this is not a wise time to make decisions. A sudden move or selling the house are decisions which should not be made overnight. Life will regain orderliness, but it is a slow process which requires much effort by the surviving loved one(s).

Sometimes, it is helpful to talk about the loss. Sometimes people find it difficult to know what to say in the face of death, so they remain silent instead of saying something inappropriate. This may be hard on the widow who needs to discuss her many mixed feelings. Widows are often excluded from social situations where, as a couple, she was formerly welcome. This may account for many widows seeking the company of other widows. This is fine as long as it does not stop the process of acceptance of the death.

Ronald J. Greer in his book, *Now That They Are Grown*, says, "I always return to the three best ways of expressing grief: cry it out, talk it out, and write it out." It is okay to cry and release those sad emotions. Find your best friend and talk about your feelings of loss and uncertainty for the future. Many people are helped by journaling. Write until you get all those emotions on paper and release them from your body. Apparently I was writing out my grief over Daddy's death when I compiled his book of letters.

Many older persons seem to almost welcome death as a friend. It frees them from their pain and suffering. This is especially true of those with a strong religious belief who view death as a release to a new and better life. **Your loved one would not want you sad and living in the past, so let it go.** Have faith that time is a great healer and get on with living your life in the best way that it can be lived.

33

Lessons to Learn

Here are some suggestions as you age.

Fulfill your dreams now. Make your wish list or bucket list and do it. Buy the diamond earrings or take that trip to Paris. Create wonderful memories! Live life to the fullest without regrets.

"Twenty years from now you will be more disappointed by the things you didn't do than by the ones you did do. So throw off the bowlines. Sail away from the safe harbor. Catch the trade winds in your sails. Explore. Dream. Discover." by Mark Twain

Take care of yourself. I like the old saying, "If I had known I was going to live this long, I would have taken better care of myself." It is never too late to exercise, eat healthy, and get seven to eight hours of sleep per night. It helps to have good genes!

Be flexible and adaptable. Make it easier for your children when it is your turn to be the aging parent. Ask your children what would make life better for them.

Be open to new possibilities. I might enjoy people my age instead of being alone. I might enjoy making new friends. I might enjoy having others do the daily chores. I might enjoy moving where my grandchildren are. That is the mindset that we need to consider.

Make friends with younger people to keep you thinking young.

Buy long-term care insurance at a young age. You do not want to be a burden to your children. If you do not have children, you definitely need this. My grandfather spent three years in a care facility, but with people living longer that number will rise. Mom has been in care facilities for six and a half years so far.

Consider moving near a child or a support group. One friend and her husband had lived in Colorado for a few years. When her husband had a health scare, they quickly moved to the small town where she attended high school and knew many people. This is where she would have the largest support group if anything happened to her husband and would be just two hours from one daughter.

Some people are retiring to friendly retirement communities like The Villages in central Florida with warm weather, where there are planned activities for all types of people, and someone else takes care of the chores. People who move there seem to love it!

Simplify; clean out and organize your possessions. Re-cycle, re-use, donate, or sell what you no longer need or use. I am not downsizing; I am upgrading! I am keeping Mom's nicer things and selling others.

Know when it is time to downsize your belongings and give up the house and yard. Depending on your health and mental condition, consider moving to senior independent living or assisted living about age 85. You want to move while you can make good decisions, while you get to choose where you move with your children's blessings, and while your mind is sharp enough to make new friends. This move is imperative when you stop driving.

Document your family history/genealogy.

Keep the family heirlooms, if possible, and document them, like the seventh generation chair and the sixth generation watch. Your children might not appreciate family heirlooms now, but their feelings might change after they reach 30, after their grandparents' deaths, or after they marry and have their own children.

Add a trustworthy person's name to your checking account.

Have your bills set up with automatic drafts.

Keep the beneficiary names current on all your assets.

Make a will or trust and living will; give a trustworthy person power of attorney. Should a church, college, or your favorite non-profit get some or all of your money? Ask your lawyer what changes should be made to your assets, such as adding Joint Ownership or Right of Survivorship. Minimize the inheritance taxes.

Document the disbursement of your belongings not covered in the will.

Document your funeral and burial wishes. Buy your burial plot and your headstone.

Write your obituary; otherwise you are at the mercy of what someone else will say about you!

Plan your finances well. Think long-term. Since my grandmothers lived to be 94 and 95, I told my financial planner I am on a 100-year plan. He had never heard anyone say they planned to live to 100. Several people in Mom's church and her facility have lived to be over 100. With people living to be older, we need to plan our finances to last as long as we do.

I like the Irish saying:

"May you never want as long as you live, and

May you live as long as you want."

When you move into an assisted living or skilled care facility:

- Sell the diamonds, fine jewelry, and furs or give them to relatives or friends to enjoy.

- Take your favorite possessions and limit the number.

Find ways to be happy now. Do not expect your children to provide your happiness.

When you help other people, it helps you more. Do random acts of kindness. It does not cost anything to say a kind word to someone.

Forgive others quickly!

Attitude is everything! Be happy where you are. I heard about a blind woman who was moving into a senior center. When someone asked about the move before she even got to her room, she said she knew she would like it. Attitude is probably the most important word in the English language.

Live the life you want and not what others want.

Stay in touch with your family and friends. Tell them you love and value them.

Use and share your talents.

How do you want to be remembered? Think about your legacy! What do you want to accomplish with that "dash" between your birth year and your death year, 19xx – 20xx?

34

Help for Elders

Ask your family doctor if he or she knows people who could stay in the home with your parents.

The Eldercare Locator is a free public service of the U.S. Administration on Aging. Call 1-800-677-1116 to speak with a specialist about programs that provide financial, employment, legal, and care giving assistance for seniors.

Some major companies, such as IBM, have Eldercare services as a part of their benefits package. Check with your company.

If your parents are veterans, see Veterans Administration Benefits: http://www.va.gov/landing2_vetsrv.htm

Consumer Consortium on Assisted Living: www.ccal.org

Several states have organizations to assist seniors. Missouri has Department of Health and Senior Services. Several states have a Division of Aging. Check your state government listing.

Compare Nursing Homes: www.medicare.gov/NHCompare

Senior daycare is provided by Sarah Care: www.sarahcare.com

Visiting Angels are in-home care providers: www.visitingangels.com

Locate a professional geriatric care manager to help find the right facility: www.caremanager.org

Information on being a resident and caregiver at The National Consumer Voice for Long-Term Care: www.theconsumervoice.org

Find valuable information about care giving and Alzheimer's disease on the Alzheimer's Association website: www.alz.org

Find Alzheimer's disease information on the National Institute on Aging website: www.alzheimers.org

Find information on dementia:
www.helpguide.org/elder/alzheimers_dementias_types.htm

Find dementia information on the National Institute on Aging website: www.dementiacarecentral.com

Find information on diseases at the Mayo Clinic's website:
http://www.mayoclinic.com/Health-Information/

Find information on diseases and care giving at
the John Hopkins' website:
http://www.johnshopkinshealthalerts.com/symptoms_remedies/

Information on Medicare: www.medicare.gov

Information on Medicaid: www.medicaid.gov

Top 5 Regrets of the Dying by Bronnie Ware:
http://www.inspirationandchai.com/Regrets-of-the-Dying.html

10 Ways to Minimize Your Regrets at the End of Your Life: http://www.allprodad.com/top10/inspirational/10-ways-to-minimize-your-regrets-at-the-end-of-your-life/

An excellent book dealing with caregivers and dementia patients:

The 36-Hour Day: A Family Guide to Caring for People with Alzheimer Disease, Other Dementias, and Memory Loss in Later Life, 4th Edition by Peter V. Rabins and Nancy L. Mace

Educational fiction book about a person getting Alzheimer's disease written by a trained professional: *Still Alice* by Lisa Genova

Note: If you decide to visit any third-party websites using links from this book, you do so at your own risk.

35

Closing

Life is about choices and consequences. Choose wisely. Choose happiness. Make the best choices for your aging parents and you to optimize your lives and to minimize the consequences. If the conditions change, you can change your choice because you get "do-overs"! (The only decision that cannot be re-done is the selling of the family home and belongings.)

Live life, so you have no regrets.

Always remember there is a beautiful young person trying to get out of that old body.

"Although the world is full of suffering, it is full also of the overcoming of it." by Helen Keller

The past is history; the future is a mystery. **All we have is now** which is why it is called the **present.**

"The past is gone. The future is not here. Now I am free of both. What am I choosing right now? **Choose joy**." Prayer by Deepak Chopra

The only definite time is **now**, so enjoy your time with your parents, your family, and your friends!

"What you feed will grow." by Bishop T. D. Jakes

Feed your thoughts with joy, happiness, peace, health, and prosperity.

Mom cannot have any expensive things at the assisted living and skilled care facilities. She has limited trips outside. If there is anything you want to enjoy, do it now. That is why I treated myself to a vacation last year. I want to create all the memories I can!

"If you had a friend you knew you'd never see again, what would you say? If you could do one last thing for someone you love, what would it be? Say it! Do it! Don't wait. **Nothing lasts forever.**" One Tree Hill, TV Show Finale

As one friend said, **"<u>Fill up on life now.</u>"**

As another friend said, **"<u>Finish well.</u>"**

You will make mistakes in caring for your parents. Just do your best and make sure your heart is truly loving and sincere.

Matthew 25:21 *"His master said to him, 'Well done, good and faithful servant....'"*

About Paula Edwards Berryann

Paula Edwards Berryann grew up in De Soto, Missouri, a small railroad town fifty miles south of St. Louis. Her family moved to Sedalia, Missouri, where she graduated from Smith-Cotton High School as Salutatorian and Outstanding Senior Girl. Paula graduated from the University of Missouri-Columbia with a Bachelor of Arts degree in mathematics, a teaching certificate, and a General Honors Certificate. She was initiated into Phi Beta Kappa, Pi Mu Epsilon (Math Honorary), and Pi Lambda Theta (Education Honorary) and was selected as one of the top fifty women in the University. While working for IBM in Poughkeepsie, NY, she attended Master's degree classes at Union College. She later transferred with IBM to Raleigh, NC, where she was a manager for fourteen years in Test, Information Systems, and Software Development and was promoted to Site Technical Education Manager. She earned two IBM Management Excellence Awards and a Teamwork Award plus attended a Division Recognition Event before taking early retirement from IBM. She was a Project Manager at PDR for several IBM manual contracts. Paula worked for OAO Technology Solutions initially as a recruiter, then as Southeast District Manager and Business Operations Manager. She returned to IBM in three supplemental assignments.

She attends Highland United Methodist Church and is active in many Mission projects. She has visited all fifty States in the United States and nine countries. Her hobbies are tennis, volleyball, traveling, reading, piano, and crocheting.

Paula compiled her Navy Seabee father's almost 700 letters to his wife into the 684 page book, *Every Thought of You, A Sailor's Love Letters from the Pacific World War II*, by Paul L. Edwards.

She has one son, Bruce, who lives in Raleigh, NC.

ALSO BY Paul L. Edwards

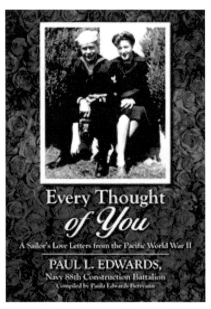

Every Thought of You

Paul L. Edwards instilled in his daughter that she could do anything she wanted. He taught her to work hard and play hard. Paula graduated Phi Beta Kappa from the University of Missouri and joined IBM, where she was a manager for many years before taking early retirement. After Paula found her father's World War II letters, she realized they showed her father's love for his wife, and their love created her. So to complete the circle of love Paula compiled all her father's World War II letters as a lasting tribute in "Every Thought of You". Women and men of all ages, lovers, baby boomers, history buffs, and military families will enjoy reading this book of love letters Paul L. Edwards wrote to his bride from training camps and the South Pacific during World War II. They were married November 27, 1941, in Sedalia, Missouri, and on December 7th the Japanese attacked Pearl Harbor. One year later Paul, a blacksmith who worked for Missouri Pacific Railroad, enlisted in the Navy 88th Construction Battalion

("Seabees") to fight the Japanese and wrote Catherine almost 700 letters, postcards, wires, and V-mail's from December, 1942, to June, 1945. These letters came from Boot Camp in Davisville, RI, two camps in California, and six islands in the South Pacific. After the Marines secured a new island in the South Pacific, Paul's Battalion moved in and built airstrips, roads, and naval bases. Paul belonged to the Masonic Lodge and believed in God, country, and brotherhood. He became an active Christian during Boot Camp. These letters of Paul's true life experiences exemplify: his patriotism and sacrifices to fight the Japanese who attacked U.S. soil in Hawaii, his love for his wife, his values, the hardships of war on sailors, their families, and friends, and the enlisted sailor's view.

These letters are a piece of history. Always remember the seventh of December! Ten percent of the author's royalties will be donated to Kansas University Endowment, Kansas City, KS, for Parkinson's disease research.

Learn more at:
www.outskirtspress.com/everythoughtofyou

CPSIA information can be obtained
at www.ICGtesting.com
Printed in the USA
BVHW041443010920
587371BV00009B/183